Turning the Tide of Male Juvenile Delinquency

Lawrence C. Grebstein, PhD, ABPP, was professor of psychology at the University of Rhode Island (URI), where his career spanned 42 years (1964–2006). He is a diplomate in clinical psychology of the American Board of Professional Psychology. At URI, he directed the Psychological Consultation Center and was director of the PhD program in clinical psychology. He was a visiting professor at the University of Bergen, Norway, and a Fellow at the Center for Family Research, George Washington University Medical Center. Dr. Grebstein has been the primary clinical psychology consultant to Ocean Tides since it began in 1975. He was in part-time private practice for 40 years. In 2006, he received the Merenda-Musiker Award of the Rhode Island Psychological Association. He has edited a book titled *Toward Self-Understanding: Studies in Personality and Adjustment*, and has written a number of professional journal articles and book chapters on family therapy and other topics. He received his BA from Brown University (1958) and his MA (1961) and PhD (1964) from the University of Kentucky. In 2013, he became a member of the affiliate medical staff at South County Hospital in the Behavioral Health Department, where he works with cancer patients in the Survivor Training and Rehabilitation (STAR) program as a volunteer.

Judy A. Van Wyk, PhD, is associate professor in the Department of Sociology and Anthropology at the University of Rhode Island, where she teaches courses in criminology, juvenile delinquency, family violence, terrorism, white-collar crime, general sociology, and social research methods. Professor Van Wyk is a productive researcher in the areas of family violence and white-collar crime, and an expert in the construction and analysis of large databases. She has published several articles in peer-reviewed journals, and book chapters that appear in edited editions. Her work is cited often in the top professional journals in criminology and criminal justice. She received her BA from the University of Oklahoma (1993), and her MA (1995) and PhD (1999) from the University of Tennessee.

Turning the Tide of Male Juvenile Delinquency

The Ocean Tides Approach

Lawrence C. Grebstein, PhD, ABPP
Judy A. Van Wyk, PhD

SPRINGER PUBLISHING COMPANY
NEW YORK

Springer Publishing Company, LLC
11 West 42nd Street
New York, NY 10036
www.springerpub.com

Acquisitions Editor: Stephanie Drew
Composition: Newgen KnowledgeWorks

ISBN: 978-0-8261-2897-3
e-book ISBN: 978-0-8261-2909-3

15 16 17 18 19/ 5 4 3 2 1

Library of Congress Cataloging-in-Publication Data
Grebstein, Lawrence C.
Turning the tide of male juvenile delinquency : the Ocean Tides approach / Lawrence C. Grebstein, Ph.D., ABPP, Judy A. Van Wyk, Ph.D.
pages cm
ISBN 978-0-8261-2897-3
1. Juvenile delinquency—Rhode Island. 2. Juvenile delinquents—Rehabilitation—Rhode Island. 3. Juvenile detention homes—Rhode Island. I. Van Wyk, Judy A. II. Ocean Tides (Rhode Island) III. Title.
HV9105.R4G74 2015
364.360811'09745—dc23 2015012474

Printed in the United States of America by McNaughton & Gunn.

To my loving family—Ellen, Ari, Laurie, Lily, Kyle, and Sheldon—and to the dedicated staff of Ocean Tides: past, present, and future.

Lawrence C. Grebstein

To my daughter Allyson and her husband Justin, who learned as much as I did from this research, whether they wanted to or not; to all of our hardworking research assistants; to my coauthor, colleague, and most importantly my friend Larry Grebstein, who trusted me with his magnum opus; and to the Ocean Tides boys, who inspire compassion and resilience in all of us.

Judy A. Van Wyk

Contents

Preface

This book is about troubled and troublesome adolescents. They have broken laws of sufficient seriousness to merit being sentenced to a youth prison or training school, but instead have been temporarily placed in a rehabilitative school for delinquent boys in Rhode Island. It is about a school called Ocean Tides that has evolved into a model educational and rehabilitative program for juveniles. This book exemplifies a multidisciplinary approach toward solving social problems through research and practice.

The authors cull information from sociology, psychology, criminology, and criminal justice to explain why juveniles commit crimes and to develop strategies toward rehabilitation that directly address the causes. Analyzing data that span 31 years from a large study of youthful offenders, they describe how the program, its design, and implementation provide a viable alternative to youth prison.

Adolescents commit crimes as a way of relieving strain in their lives that is created by the presence of negative experiences and by the absence of positive and constructive parenting, resulting in the imbalance of reinforcements over constraints against criminal coping. For the most part, delinquents are just kids who, by virtue of circumstances that are usually beyond their own control, make the wrong choices. Rehabilitating youthful offenders requires changing these circumstances: taking them away from those negative experiences, providing supportive surrogate parenting, helping them to realize their own potential, and emphasizing their own talents and strengths to guide them away from crime.

The focus of the book is on how to help young men, who have gone sufficiently astray to be incarcerated, change their lives for the better. We describe a residential education and treatment program that began in the mid-1970s and at the time was a nontraditional way of dealing with court-adjudicated male juvenile delinquents. The national trend, beginning in the late 1970s, was toward a more punitive orientation in contrast to rehabilitation in the 1960s. The new trend involved harsher and longer sentences and trying more juveniles as adults, and continued through the 1980s to the early 1990s. In 1993 and 1994 there were spikes in violent crime among juveniles that were primarily due to demographic changes in the population structure brought on by the coming of age of the second generation of baby boomers. Nonetheless, this crime spike reinforced and strengthened the punitive approach. Researchers and practitioners warned of the ill effects that incarcerating juveniles had on them and began offering assistance to states to reform their juvenile justice systems. For example, "since 1992, the Juvenile Detention Alternatives Initiative, a project of the Annie E. Casey Foundation, has demonstrated that jurisdictions can safely reduce reliance on secure confinement and generally strengthen their juvenile justice systems through a series of interrelated reform strategies" (Annie E. Casey Foundation, 2014). However, rather than questioning the utility of a punitive approach, the emphasis on punishment intensified, and this national trend continued at least until 2004. The sharp decline in crime that followed the spike in the 1990s was incorrectly attributed to the effectiveness of the punitive approach by some policy makers. As youth detention facilities began to burst at the seams around 2005 and recidivism skyrocketed to 85%, state officials began to examine alternatives to incarceration. Now they seem to be running in the opposite direction and many policy makers are leaning toward home confinement for troubled teens in an effort to save money. Unfortunately, confining a delinquent to the very environment that may have produced the initial problems in the first place will only result in more criminal behavior right into adulthood. Incarceration and home confinement are extreme reactions to juvenile crime and neither one makes sense, but there are logical and proven alternatives to these extremes.

The goals of this book are to provide useful empirical information about male juvenile delinquents; to serve as a model training manual for new programs and people working in existing rehabilitation programs; to provide guidelines for developing policy on the rehabilitation of juvenile delinquents; to be a resource for academicians and others who teach courses on juvenile delinquency; and to be assigned as a supplementary textbook for students learning about juvenile delinquency, juvenile justice, and mental health.

CONTRIBUTIONS TO THE LITERATURE

Research Methods

The Ocean Tides project is the first of its kind. It is first to amass comprehensive data on juvenile delinquents from so many different sources. Rich sources provided the researchers the ability to check and cross-check information about the boys for accuracy. The juvenile justice community that includes practitioners, clinicians, researchers, and educators has long predicted that delinquents would fare much better in rehabilitative diversionary programs than in youth prisons or in home confinement. However, to date, there is no study that empirically tests the validity of this assumption on a large database of delinquents with information derived from a plethora of sources about these young men's characteristics, behaviors, and experiences. Studies that do include analyses of empirical data on juvenile delinquents do not access multiple sources, as these authors do. They instead typically focus on one of the two sources for information: (a) police records or (b) self-reports from the juveniles. Juveniles commit an average of five serious crimes before they are officially arrested in the United States. A juvenile may have been arrested for burglary but have a long history of violent behavior that is missed in studies that limit their data to police records. Hence, in these studies, juveniles are being misclassified. This study finds that nearly 5% of violent juveniles would have been misclassified as nonviolent had it relied solely on police records.

Research on juveniles indicates that self-reports of misbehavior are equally unreliable because respondents tend to overexaggerate some types of crimes and underreport others. Compounding the problem, several self-report studies on juveniles use telephone-survey methods, and parental supervision during the interviews restricts honest disclosure, especially about violent victimization that may be going on at home. Using multiple sources of information about the boys' behaviors and their experiences allowed the researchers to check and cross-check information for the most accurate analyses. No other study exists that has taken this approach to create a large database—partly because it is typically costly and time-consuming to do—but these authors have done it.

Family Violence Literature

One of the several important findings from the research is that nearly 58% of the Ocean Tides boys behaved violently prior to entering the program and that figure drops to 22% while residing in the program. Prior to entering the Ocean Tides program, boys who were physically or sexually abused, or boys who were exposed to physical violence among parental figures, were most likely to act violently versus strictly engaging in nonviolent forms of behavior. Once boys were in the Ocean Tides program, the effects of prior physical and sexual abuse on violence are diminished, and the effects of exposure to parental interpersonal violence (PIPV) on violent behavior at Ocean Tides disappear. These findings challenge commonly held assumptions in the family violence literature that the effects of exposure to PIPV on future violent behavior may be permanent.

Contributions to Theory of Family Therapy

Agnew's General Theory of Crime

This is one of the first tests of Agnew's general theory of crime that focuses on strains that are produced from within families even though the family domain is the most influential component of this theory. This is a criminological theory that explains how and why people who experience the same events can respond differently. It is very helpful for practitioners working in the mental health profession to broaden their scope of understanding and look to fields outside of psychology that may provide them with more tools to use when counseling juvenile offenders.

Family Therapy Theories

The description of the program illustrates the use and application to delinquency of an integrative eclectic model of family counseling and evaluation that incorporates aspects of structural family therapy, problem-centered systems therapy of the family, and strategic family therapy. This approach hones the most effective strategies into a single unified evolutionary approach to rehabilitation.

HOW THE BOOK CAN BE USED

The authors of this book take a multidisciplinary approach that will appeal to everyone who thinks about juvenile delinquency: politicians; judges; police; teachers; clinicians; social workers; educators; and students of criminology, criminal justice, juvenile delinquency, family violence, sociology, psychology, and counseling. This approach appeals to undergraduate students in liberal arts programs that require them to take courses in multiple disciplines, and to graduate students in the mental health fields whose undergraduate training varies.

This book provides information that can be used as a guide to develop a juvenile rehabilitation program for delinquents from the ground up, or depending on the reader's needs, it can be used to strengthen some component of an existing program. Regardless of who the reader is or what role that person plays in rehabilitating juvenile offenders, there is something in this book for everyone.

Informing Juvenile Justice Reform

The book merges some of the hottest topics that currently grip the attention of Americans: the mental health of juvenile delinquents, criminal justice expenditures, families, education, and violence. This trend has generated changes in the juvenile justice system, causing many states, like Rhode Island, to search for less expensive and more effective alternatives to incarcerating juveniles. This study helps to specify which types of programs may work best to rehabilitate juvenile delinquents, and it provides a how-to guide for structuring these initiatives.

Informing Future Research

Taking an empirically based approach to juvenile justice reform, this research can inform future studies and provide rationale for more careful methods that lead to more valid results. In the rush to publish or perish in academia, excellence in research often suffers. Funding agencies are reluctant to pay for projects as large and time-consuming as this undertaking was. This study exemplifies how careful and targeted research methods yield the most accurate and useful results.

As a Secondary Text for Undergraduates and Graduate Students

As a secondary text for undergraduate students, this book provides the next best thing to a hands-on practicum with juvenile delinquents. It allows students to see the theories that they learn about from primary texts coming to life. It is easy to read and follow. It also provides practical skills for interviewing juvenile delinquents that can be practiced in the classroom. This book will be very useful to students taking courses in psychology, counseling, sociology, criminology, policing, law, social work, family violence, and public policy. Furthermore, the book is useful to students doing internships in programs like Ocean Tides, and it should be read before participating in these programs.

The book can be used for both theory and practice courses in clinical psychology, social work, counseling, marital and family therapy, and criminal justice. Students doing externships working with delinquents and adult prisoners will also find it helpful.

As a Training Manual for Practitioners

Designing and implementing an effective rehabilitation program for juvenile delinquents is no easy matter. It involves an educational component, life skills training, increasing interpersonal skills, developing vocational skills and good work habits, and improving self-esteem and self-efficacy. Eliminating antisocial and other disruptive behavior requires not only careful planning but considerable trial-and-error implementation over time to see what works. The description of the procedures developed in this program provides useful and practical guidelines for anyone working with delinquents and other young men engaging in disruptive behavior.

PRACTICAL TIPS FOR PRACTITIONERS

This book offers practical tips for practitioners at every level of the development and implementation of reform in juvenile rehabilitation programming. For policy makers and state legislators, it offers practical rationales for developing these programs and uses empirically based evidence of their effectiveness. The book provides a complete description of each component of a successful program for delinquents that state-level juvenile justice commissions can model. Likewise, policy makers learn how much money can be saved in juvenile justice expenditures by developing programs like Ocean Tides, and how these programs ultimately decrease demands on the adult correctional system by lowering rates of recidivism.

Program organizers and administrators will learn about potential political hurdles they may confront in developing an effective rehabilitative or educational program for delinquents. They will learn how each component of a good program should work—the rationale, philosophies, and reasons for each component of the program. Finally, this research underscores the fact that simply removing a child from a bad household may not be enough. Furthermore, these juveniles need functional surrogate parents who foster corrective emotional experiences, and this book explains what a program like that should contain.

Every chapter in this book provides tips for mental health professionals and for program consultants. Treatment methods and prevention programs that are developed by clinical counselors need to be guided by a broad-based theoretical understanding of why juveniles commit crimes. This involves identifying patterns of trauma that predate the delinquent behavior, such as family violence. These experiences create strain in a child's life that must be relieved before further treatment can be effective. Social workers and Department of Children,Youth and Families employees often conduct home visits and can spot signs of parental violence and child abuse, but only if they are aware of their dangers.

This book provides detailed information about how these programs should be structured and what they can offer. Consultants who are hired to design specific components of a program can use the descriptions in this book as a model for program design. They will learn how their work will fit into the overall program design and philosophy. Consultants can learn what they can do to improve the functioning of programs that already exist. The book details their roles and responsibilities, and provides a how-to guide for providing in-service training, moderating staff meetings, conducting workshops, mediating conflicts and disagreements among staff, advising and consulting administrators and department heads, and evaluating administrators. The book provides how-to strategies for developing more successful communication strategies with delinquents so that mental health providers can detect and prevent problems such as suicide or violent behavior, and prescribe more targeted medications. They can obtain real information directly from their delinquent clients that is accurate for guiding rehabilitation and treatment strategies. They can get valid information from clients about what is going on at home to provide more effective outpatient counseling. Finally, this book provides real-life stories that help practitioners to see the potential outcomes of a program like Ocean Tides.

Staff members who are already working in rehabilitation programs can learn what the overall goals should be for these programs and learn about how their different efforts fit into the larger whole. Staff in different parts of the program will learn what their roles are and how to do their jobs most effectively within the whole system. Staff members who work with delinquents can use these strategies to reduce conflict.

Police who read this book will benefit from learning about delinquent boys, what their families are like, and their characteristics, in order to understand how to deal with them. For example, a lot of the Ocean Tides boys hope to grow up and be police officers themselves, which could potentially place the officer in a mentoring relationship with young offenders. Police need to understand that young offenders are often also victims of abuse. Exposure to PIPV is child abuse, and children should be removed from these abusive situations not only for their own safety but also to prevent subsequent delinquency. Police can use the communication strategies that are explained in the book to minimize disorderly conduct and conflict during arrest because they often inadvertently incite these problems through their miscommunication with delinquents.

Family court judges need to know what a program has to offer before they know who would benefit the most from the programs they have to offer, and they need to know what works best. They typically make the decision where to place a juvenile delinquent, so it is imperative that they are able to identify and recognize effective components of a rehabilitation program in order to make the best decision possible for the delinquent.

This book provides researchers with a clear explanation of the study methods, and describes the database and its construction so that other researchers may be guided by example. Researchers will also benefit from learning how to interview delinquents to foster more valid information. Researchers learn the benefits of using multiple sources of information on juvenile delinquents. For example, this research finds that nearly 5% of violent juveniles would have been incorrectly categorized as nonviolent in the research if only arrest records were used to measure violence.

Anyone who comes in contact with children at school—teachers, nurses, and counselors—needs to increase awareness about the dangers of child abuse and exposure to PIPV. If a child acts out at school, the adults there need to recognize that exposure to PIPV may be involved. Teachers can learn a lot from this book about how to detect and develop strengths that children possess and may not even understand themselves. These strategies can even be used to minimize class disruptions and to foster effective learning at school.

A SYNOPSIS OF WHAT FOLLOWS

Chapter 1—Ocean Tides Rising: History

The first chapter in the book is a brief history of juvenile delinquency in the United States and in Rhode Island from the 1850s until the establishment of the Ocean Tides program in 1975. The discussion chronicles the events and policies, both nationally and locally, that shaped and characterized how juvenile delinquents were conceptualized and treated. The authors describe the specific events in Rhode Island that led to the founding of Ocean Tides.

Chapter 2—Currents: Who the Boys Are

This chapter is a description of the population in residence in the Ocean Tides program from 1975 through 2006, including the intake criteria for acceptance into the program. The authors describe the nature of the database, its development, and the sources of information used for constructing the database. The chapter contains demographic and other information about the delinquents and their families, including ethnic and racial composition of the residents and demographic changes over time; information about substance abuse, child abuse, abandonment and rejection, and the residents' and their families' criminal charges; and information about behavior and attitudes, psychological characteristics, school performance, career aspirations, and interests among the residents.

Chapter 3—Explaining the Ocean Tides: Theory

In this chapter, the authors explain why and how juveniles become delinquent. After a brief summary of criminological theory, the chapter provides a more in-depth description of Robert Agnew's general theory of crime. This includes a discussion of the major components that contribute to crime, such as cultural influences, outside factors, and strain in the five life domains. Juveniles engage in delinquency to relieve the strains brought about by exposure to violence between parental figures, child abuse (negative experiences), and the absence of positive parenting (removal of something positive) in the presence of reinforcements and minimal constraints. Through the fostering of positive relationships, the Ocean Tides program serves as surrogate parents and removes the adolescent from negative experiences at home, thus relieving at least two forms of strain that can lead to violence. Empirical evidence presented in the following chapter supports this theory.

Chapter 4—An Undertow: Personal Child Abuse Victimization and Exposure to Parental Interpersonal Violence

In Chapter 4, the authors explore the role of family and the effects of domestic violence in contributing to the development of delinquent behavior. In particular, the discussion focuses on the long-term effects of exposure to

PIPV and how it contributes to the development of violent behavior in the young men. The authors review several shortcomings in the existing research on exposure to PIPV; describe how this is the first study to test the long-term effects of PIPV using information from multiple sources; and describe how the ill effects of exposure can be ameliorated by removing the youngster from the family and placing him in a supportive program while family relationships are strengthened through counseling.

Chapter 5—Charting a Course: The Program at Ocean Tides

Chapter 5 provides a description of the Ocean Tides program and its three main components: the school, social services department, and supervision of residential life. In addition to describing the organization and administration of the program, the authors discuss the role of the treatment teams, staff and their roles and duties, and how the program works on a daily basis.

Chapter 6—Calming Seas: Managing the Ocean Tides Residents

Chapter 6 provides additional information about how the Ocean Tides program works. Information includes the underlying treatment philosophies (Reality Therapy and the LaSallian Heritage) and detailed descriptions of the various interventions used by teachers, social services counselors, and residential staff. The authors describe how special programs, such as anger management, social skills training, and sexual offender treatment, are integrated into the program. Relevant data from the research project are integrated into the discussion.

Chapter 7—Navigating the Waters: The Role of the Clinical Psychologist as a Consultant

In this chapter, the authors explain how a clinical psychologist can be used as a consultant to the program and how this role changes as a program develops. Specific functions include staff support and supervision;

leading and moderating full staff meetings; providing in-service training and workshops; mediating conflicts and disagreements among staff; contributing to staff development of policy and procedures; conducting interview-based psychological evaluations of residents; and conducting annual evaluations of department heads and other administrators.

Chapter 8—At the Helm: Interviewing Adolescent Male Juvenile Delinquents

In the eighth chapter, the authors describe key issues and difficulties associated with conducting evaluation interviews with delinquent boys, including how to evaluate suicidal potential and risk of violent behavior. The authors discuss both underlying philosophy and specific techniques involved in interviewing and describe a "curiosity model" of interviewing. They explain that the interview is integral to establishing trusting relationships with delinquents and is necessary for directing rehabilitation strategies that are specific to the juvenile's needs.

Chapter 9—Stem the Tide: Case Histories

Chapter 9 includes case histories of six of the Ocean Tides residents along with a couple of the students' essays written in their own words about their own lives. It provides a unique glimpse into the personal triumphs and obstacles these boys have faced in their young lives.

Chapter 10—Sailing Home: Final Thoughts

This chapter summarizes the main focuses of the research and the book and identifies its significant conclusions. A section in this chapter is devoted to explaining what changes have occurred at Ocean Tides since 2007, and policy and research strategies are discussed.

REFERENCE

Annie E. Casey Foundation. (2014). Juvenile Detention Alternatives Initiative (Web Page). Retrieved from http://www.aecf.org/work/juvenile-justice/jdai/

Acknowledgments

Many persons have contributed to the successful completion of this book. The research project was supported in part by two grants from the U.S. Department of Justice, Office of Juvenile Justice and Delinquency Prevention. The Rhode Island Juvenile Justice Advisory Committee awarded the grants. The authors are indebted to the Committee and to Elizabeth Gilheeney, juvenile justice specialist, for her invaluable help in the application process and administration of these grants. Br. Joseph Schafer, FSC, former director of social services, was indispensable in helping the authors and research assistants with locating and managing the clinical files for the research project. He also read an early draft of the manuscript and provided helpful feedback. Br. Brendan Gerrity, FSC, president and director of Ocean Tides for the past 33 years, gave his complete support to the research project. The following persons provided information in their respective areas and/or read portions of the manuscript to ensure accurate reporting of information: Norah Sargent, PhD, consultant in clinical psychology and director of the Sexual Offender Program; Jane Genereux, principal of Ocean Tides School; Charles Coutu, assistant principal in charge of the Providence Campus; Ryan Carreau, vice president and director of residential living; Deb McCurdy, director of social services; Celine Johnson, director of special education; Gary Comunale, director of vocational training; Br. John McGann, FSC, court liaison; Andy Lussier, executive chef and director of the culinary arts program; Rich Lemieux, wood-turning teacher; Rich Soderberg, woodshop teacher; Nancy Lyon, art teacher; and Brian Sullivan, director of administration. The important and tedious work of coding the information from the clinical files to the database was accomplished by the following undergraduate and graduate students (indicated by GS after their names) from the University of Rhode Island, who worked either for academic credit or, in some cases, as paid research assistants: Amanda Alfano, Cara Baccoli, Leslie Barber, Lisa Basiliere, Ryan Batalon, Nicole Bedard, Josh Board, Maria Cambio, Michael Cecchini, Shabnam Danesh, Kristen Degregorio, Erin Devaney, Eric Scott Endres, Kara Eriksen (GS), Wayne Everheart, Sandra Faria, Angelina Franciosa, Grisel M. Garcia (GS), Marissa Goldstein, Felicia Gomes, Aaron Goodpasture, Daniel Hughes, Graham Johnson, Jeremy Jordan, Aliza Langman Krieger (GS), Felicia Walker Lospaluto, Silvermoon Mars, Courtney McCarthy, Kaitlyn McManus, Hayley Nemiroff, Kristen Nunes, Damian Puerini, Allyson Van Wyk Quintanilla, Justin Quintanilla, Marshall Robinson (GS), Christine Sapienza, Kristen Scott, Erin Thornton, Taryn Valpey, Sheila Vaughn, Melissa Wein, Amber Wells, and Melissa Zuba. Finally, Sheldon Grebstein, PhD, read several chapters of the manuscript and gave valuable feedback regarding clarity of writing and literary merit.

CHAPTER 1

Ocean Tides Rising: History

There is a tide in the affairs of men which, taken
at the flood, leads on to fortune, omitted,
all the voyage of their lives is bound in shallows
and in misery.— WILLIAM SHAKESPEARE

The term *juvenile delinquency* is not new, originating during the 1700s (Mennel, 1973), and criminal prosecution of delinquent behavior predates the phrase (Sanders, 1970). English laws in the 7th and 8th centuries specified criminal penalties for children as young as 10 or 11 years (Shoemaker, 2009). For as long as juveniles have misbehaved, official responses have evolved adjusting to political, social, economic, and pedagogical pressures.

JUVENILE DELINQUENCY IN THE UNITED STATES

In the United States, the system of juvenile-specific facilities began in the mid-1850s with the establishment of institutions variously labeled as reformatories, training schools, protectorates, or industrial schools (Shoemaker, 2009). During the latter half of the 19th century, institutions improved and became more specialized with regard to the types of children they served. In an attempt to improve services, many of these institutions employed the "cottage system." In this model, cottages housed up to 30 residents and were supervised by a pair of cottage "parents."

According to Shoemaker (2009), the cottage system reflected the correctional thinking of the time that placed the family at the center of the young persons' lives. The prevalent belief was that the family was primarily responsible for causing the juveniles' misguided behavior and the family, or a family surrogate, should be at the core of any attempts to change the behavior. By recreating the family in the form of a cottage, the juveniles' antisocial attitudes and behaviors could be changed to more socially acceptable and conforming behaviors (Shoemaker, 2009). Despite the attempt to improve services through reforms and new developments, there remained an ideological split between punishment and rehabilitation as the best approach for dealing with the incarcerated youngsters.

Guidelines for placement in the early reform schools were similar across the country and generally reflected a more punishment–reform approach.

> School trustees are empowered to receive all children under eighteen years of age as shall be convicted before any court sitting within the limits of said city as vagrants or disorderly persons or of criminal offenses committed within the limits of said city. In addition to these, any child over five years of age might also, at the request of his parent or guardian, be received in the school. All children admitted or committed to the institution were to be properly disciplined, instructed and employed until they should be reformed, discharged or bound out. (Crepeau, 1941, p. 162)

Children were sent to the court not only for criminal violations of the law, but for other reasons, such as being poor or because the parents were unable to provide appropriate care in the eyes of the court. Although these decisions were challenged in a number of litigations, the U.S. Supreme Court upheld the lower courts' rights to remove a child from his or her home through the use of the *parens patriae* principle. This doctrine states that the court can act as the "common guardian of the community" when parents are unable to take responsibility for the care and education of their children (Mennel, 1973, p. 14).

As a result of the work of a group of reformers known as "child savers," the first delinquency law and juvenile court were established in Cook County, Illinois. This law established that youngsters aged

16 years or younger were under the jurisdiction of the juvenile court. The age was later raised to 17 years for boys and 18 years for girls (Dohrn, 2002, p. 271). The establishment of this law and court set a new precedent and standard for dealing with delinquent youth that was emulated in most states. The significance of the establishment of this first juvenile court was noted by Handler and Zatz (1982, p. 21):

> The founding of the juvenile court was a milestone in juvenile justice reform. It represented the culmination of a century-long effort to rehabilitate and protect dependent, neglected, incorrigible and delinquent youth through the coercive intervention of the state for the purpose of instilling proper moral values. As such, the court became a vehicle for the child reform movement, of which the social worker, teacher and psychologist were also now an integral part. Its treatment philosophy was predicated on the assumption that children who appeared before the court were not inherently bad, but were in need of educative and purposeful activity.

According to Tanenhaus (2002, p. 45), all but two states (Maine and Wyoming) had some form of delinquency law by 1925, and all cities with a population more than 100,000 had juvenile courts.

This prevailing philosophy for dealing with juvenile delinquents shifted like a pendulum for more than 100 years between punishment and rehabilitation until a sharp spike in delinquency rates in the United States in the 1960s sparked fear in the public, and the criminal justice system had to more directly respond. As early as 1967, researchers attributed most of this rise in crime to the changing age structure of the population that resulted from the post–World War II baby boom. Between 1960 and 1965, the fastest growing proportion of the population was 15 to 24 years old (President's Commission, 1967, p. 20). The age–crime relationship is well established in criminology. "Crime flourishes when there are many restless, relatively footloose young people in the population" (President's Commission, 1967, p. 16). The most likely period in a person's life to engage in illegal behavior is while he or she is young, 12 to 24 years on average. People generally begin to age out of crime starting around 24 years or later depending on the type of crime. Likewise, victims and offenders most often share demographic characteristics, such as age. During the 1960s, America had the largest pool of potential offenders and victims of crime compared to the adult population than in any other decade prior to or since then.

Several studies conclude that a substantial amount of the 1960s' rise in crime in general and the rise in crime in the juvenile population is attributable to the age composition in the United States. Sagi and Wellford (1968) found that the age structure of the population accounted for 25% to 40% of the increases. The 1965 President's Commission on crime said, "commission studies based on 1960 arrest rates indicate that between 1960 and 1965 about 40 to 50 percent of the total increase in the arrests reported by UCR (Uniform Crime Reports) could have been expected as the result of increases in population and changes in the age composition of the population" (President's Commission, 1967, p. 28). Using more advanced statistical procedures available in the 1980s, Cohen and Land (1987) reexamined Sagi and Wellford's study and found that, accounting for the increased number of potential victims as well as offenders in the 1960s, an even greater proportion of the increase is attributed to the age structure than originally thought. Likewise, some researchers have concluded that as much as 70% of the decline in crime between 1980 and 1984 occurred because the baby boom children simply aged out of crime (Steffensmeier & Harer, 1987). Nonetheless, the public was fearful in the 1960s of the changes they were seeing in the youth culture overall, and the increase in crime garnered official reaction.

Several developments occurred in the 1960s. Congress passed the Juvenile Delinquency and Youth Offenses Act, which grew out of the President's Committee on Juvenile Delinquency and Youth Crime. This law appropriated $10 million for each year between 1962 and 1965. This money was intended to coordinate all federal programs in dealing with the problem of juvenile delinquency.

In 1965, President Johnson established the President's Commission on Law Enforcement and Administration of Justice to examine every aspect of state, local, and federal crime control. This massive effort included 19 commission members and 32 professional staff members. The Commission was divided into five major task forces that drew on the expertise of more than 300 professionals and academics to examine (a) the impacts of crime on American society, (b) improvements in policing, (c) courts, (d) corrections, probation, and parole, and (e) using science and technology to improve the overall system. Specific crime problems were addressed across all five task forces, such as organized crime and juvenile delinquency. The Commission undertook several studies to fulfill its charter and its work culminated in a final report to the president in February 1967, titled *The Challenge of Crime in a Free Society: A Report by the President's Commission on Law Enforcement and Administration of Justice*. Chapter 3 of this report titled "Juvenile Delinquency and Youth Crime" (pp. 55–89) and subsequent publications stemming from the studies conducted for this report significantly shaped juvenile crime control strategies in the United States from 1967 to 1980.

Maloney (1986, p. 51) notes: "The year 1967 was to be a major turning point for the entire juvenile justice system in the United States," in large part due to the President's Commission report that strongly criticized the juvenile justice system and called for major changes. Included in the recommendations were increased efforts toward prevention by "diverting" children from the justice system before they got into serious trouble. Labeling children as criminals alienates them from legitimate opportunities in every social institution; that is, family, education, and work. The report also questioned the effectiveness of the structurally institutional model as the primary mode of dealing with the juvenile offender. If the purpose of officially recognizing delinquent behavior was to rehabilitate children, then locking them up and separating them from society could not possibly solve the problem. The work of this task force resulted in the Juvenile Delinquency Prevent and Control Act of 1968. This law allocated $150 million to aid juvenile justice systems at the state and local levels as a complement to earlier federal dollars and to facilitate the development of new types of programs.

Another major event contributed to reforms made during the 1960s that changed the experiences of juveniles in the American criminal justice system. The Supreme Court in 1967 ruled that juveniles had the right to due process. This ruling challenged the way juvenile courts had been operating and opened the door for a major overhaul in the way the juvenile justice system operated. In 1974, Congress passed the Juvenile Justice Delinquency Prevention Act. This act emphasized the use of community-based alternatives to custodial institutions, such as diversionary programs, rehabilitative counseling services, small residential treatment centers, and community-based group homes (Maloney, 1986). From a practical point of view, the federal government provided "seed" money to the states to help start new approaches to dealing with delinquency. As a result, the private sector became involved in providing treatment for delinquents through the development of alternative programs and models.

The Situation in Rhode Island

Historically, the treatment of juvenile offenders in Rhode Island paralleled what had been happening in the rest of the country. The Providence Reform School that was established in 1850 became the central institution for juvenile criminals from the whole state because the state's population was about the same size as Boston at that time. In 1880, the state officially took over the Providence Reform School and, in 1882, opened new buildings at the state farm in Cranston, Rhode Island, a then rural community adjacent to the capital city of Providence. There were two separate schools, one for boys and one for girls, consisting of two clusters of cottages located across the road and in close proximity to each other. The Sockanosset School for boys and Oaklawn School for girls were later renamed as the Rhode Island Training Schools (for boys or girls), but, for many years, were popularly known simply as "Sockanosset" or "Oaklawn." The schools originally opened in 1882 with 138 boys and 20 girls and are still located in the same area today. The distinctive white cement and gray granite block cottages stand as an iconic warning for youngsters of what might happen to them if they misbehave. One of the authors (Grebstein) recalls the obligatory Sunday afternoon family automobile rides to the country in the 1940s and 1950s and hearing his parents warn as they passed the reform school that he might end up in Sockanosset if he did not mind them well. This threat was not unique to his family but was commonplace among families in Rhode Island with young boys.

The Rhode Island Training Schools were essentially workhouses where residents spent most of their time working in the facility's own print shop or they were farmed out for work elsewhere. By 1868, a full-scale investigation revealed serious physical and emotional abuses against residents. In 1890, a military school was instituted as part of the overall program (Field, 1902). Although the overriding philosophy at the training school was confinement and strict punishment, Rhode Island courts were beginning to reflect national pressures toward reform.

The first separate juvenile court was established in Rhode Island in 1898 but was contained within the adult court. The Rhode Island General Assembly established a probation system for juveniles in 1899. The juvenile court was formalized by the Juvenile Court Act of 1915, but was not established as a separate entity from the district court until 1944. The juvenile justice system, however, remained unchanged from the turn of the century. It consisted of three components: the reform schools, separate court proceedings for juveniles, and a probation system. In 1961, the Rhode Island General Assembly established the first family court in the United States to deal with family matters and issues related to children. Previously, all domestic issues, except for delinquency petitions, were handled in the regular court system.

Corresponding to the reform developments nationally and the actions taken by the federal government, the state formed a task force to address the rising juvenile crime rate during the early 1960s. The task force (Rhode Island Commission to Study Juvenile Delinquency) issued its report in 1965. The report provided a blueprint for changes over the subsequent 15 years. Included in the recommendations were the establishment of a new diagnostic center to assess youngsters and determine the type of treatment needed; new training schools for both boys and girls; a new family court building; improved services at the training schools with a greater emphasis on treatment rather than custody; the establishment of group homes and halfway houses for youngsters at risk; the requirement that local police departments designate certain police officers as juvenile specialists; and the creation of a school of social work at Rhode Island College to develop more trained professionals.

A new superintendent at the training school (for boys), Joseph Devine, in 1968, attempted to implement new and more progressive innovations, such as a work-release program, smaller classes in school, individual progress reports (which replaced the prison-modeled classification board), and individual and group counseling programs. Sadly, the new strategies were too disorganized to be effective. The superintendent stated:

> The institution as a whole lacked direction, purpose, and a cohesive wholeness. In my eagerness to change the brutal, dehumanizing institution that I found into a force for rehabilitation, I had embraced any and all programs that came along. I was willing to let anyone try almost anything. I had no critical standards against which to measure what we were doing. As a result the institution suffered from an aimless drift. (Carkhuff, 1974, p. 4)

Before the new superintendent's arrival, the cottage managers ran the school and the residents. They perceived the new superintendent and his reforms as a threat. Their status was the primary source of their job satisfaction. As they saw their authority and influence diminishing, they gave up completely, longing for the "good old days" when toughness and order prevailed. The residents exploited this passivity, resulting in riots in 1969.

In response to the riots, the superintendent enlisted professional help from Robert Carkhuff, PhD, who was responsible for the human resource development model that the correctional counseling programs in the Federal Bureau of Prisons was using (Carkhuff, 1974). Carkhuff and Devine called the new program "Operation Changeover."

The existing staff for this new program underwent intense training and new staff were handpicked so that they were more responsive to the new approaches. For residents, Operation Changeover focused on interpersonal development and was oriented toward individual care. The program reached beyond the boys' confinement in the institution and implemented a family outreach program. The program was fully implemented in 1971.

The new approach appeared to be succeeding when a new political appointee, Department of Corrections Director Anthony Travisano, abruptly fired the superintendent in 1972 over alleged labor-hiring violations. Following this, the institution returned to its former highly structured and custodial orientation. According to Carkhuff (1974), the results were disastrous.

> A once proud institution hung her head in shame. Riots broke out in the cottages. A cottage master was stabbed. Racial strife intensified. Break-ins and burglaries within the institution increased dramatically. The runaway rate mushroomed. In the first three months following the dismantling of "Changover," 109 students were on elopement status. (p. vii)

The situation continued to deteriorate. Maloney (1986) summarized the state of treatment and rehabilitation for juvenile delinquents in Rhode Island at that time as follows:

> Although a great deal of good work had been done to design an effective system of probation, to bring reform to the State Training school and to effect more preventive and

> treatment-oriented programs for Rhode Island's juvenile offenders during the 1960's, the reality of early 1970's seemed to indicate a more fragmented and ineffective system than ever existed in previous years. As the United States Congress passed the Juvenile Justice Delinquency Prevention Act in 1974, Rhode Island's system appeared to be in a serious crisis and few other alternatives existed that could offer services to delinquent youth in the State. (pp. 94–95)

THE FOUNDING OF THE OCEAN TIDES PROGRAM

The situation in Rhode Island with regard to the treatment of juvenile offenders was ripe for change and the introduction of new approaches. At the height of the crisis in the state's programs for juvenile delinquency, two Christian brothers with extensive experience in working with delinquents, Br. Robert Wagner and Br. Michael Reis, were investigating various delinquency programs in the Northeast looking for new opportunities. Both men had worked at Lincoln Hall, a large facility for juvenile delinquents in New York. Br. Robert, a professor of criminal justice at the John Jay School, had 24 years of experience, and Br. Michael, a prison chaplain, had 6 years' experience. Both men were looking for a less institutional and more innovative program. Providing services for troubled youngsters was not a new vocation for men within this order.

The Brothers of the Christian Schools (hereafter referred to as the Christian Brothers) are a group of Roman Catholic men who have been dedicated to teaching and education work since their founding in the 17th century by Saint John Baptist de La Salle. The Christian Brothers have a long tradition of dealing with troubled youth and juvenile offenders dating back to the early 1700s. In 1705, Saint LaSalle started a school for juvenile delinquents in Rouen, France (Battersby, 1970). They continued this work after establishing themselves in the United States in 1846 (Gabriel, 1948). They involved themselves with the education and care of youngsters who were poor, delinquent, orphaned, and from working middle-class parents. Maloney (1986), citing Battersby (1970), lists 11 different institutions in the eastern and midwestern United States that were founded by the Christian Brothers between 1853 and 1906 to provide services to these disenfranchised youngsters. They had been in Rhode Island since 1871 and had established several schools. One school in particular, LaSalle Academy, an academic preparatory high school in Providence, had an influential impact on the state by producing a number of graduates who went on to pursue important careers in law, politics, and the state judiciary.

Maloney (1986), in an interview with Br. Michael Reis, identified several factors that contributed to the creation of the Ocean Tides program. A great deal of change was occurring in the field of juvenile justice in the United States. For example, the neighboring state of Massachusetts had recently closed all of its training schools and deinstitutionalization was the latest trend. In his role as a chaplain at the adult prison in Rhode Island, Br. Michael became familiar with the problems facing the troubled youth. Finally, the former novitiate of the province was empty and available. The Christian Brothers had closed the program in 1969 because of the declining number of new novices entering the vocation. The novitiate was a beautiful building with 60 bedrooms located on 10 acres in Narragansett, Rhode Island, directly across from the ocean. Lindner and Wagner (1983, p. 26) describe the setting:

> The splendors of a past age, including richly carved mahogany paneled conference rooms and oversized fireplaces, are still visible and provide a tone of quiet dignity, often in sharp contrast to the institutional furnishings so typically found in juvenile institutions. Neither would one expect to find a juvenile center situated in the midst of the idyllic surrounding on which the ten-acre site is located. The property overlooks the Narragansett Bay in Rhode Island in an area renowned as a summer resort area. Surrounded by equally impressive mini-estates, one marvels both at the scenic beauty and the incongruity of the site as a juvenile institution. The natural beauty of the area is, however, seen as a positive force in the overall treatment process. From its start, Ocean Tides has worked from the premise that the physical surrounds...are an integral part of climate; they are important and formative context for interpersonal programmatic treatment efforts.

It was an ideal setting for a new residential program for delinquents. Br. Louis DeThomasis, then vice president for finance for his brothers' province, vividly describes the origins of what eventually grew into Ocean Tides.

> I thought they were dreaming. When Mike (Br. Michael Reis) first brought up the idea of a program for delinquents. I never paid him much mind. Sure he could use the building! At that point, the former novitiate was seldom used and was deteriorating. It was costing us more and more money and was one big headache when simply viewed as an idle structure and as a bleak reminder of the changing times. But then suddenly one day, I realized they were serious about this program. Both men knew kids, especially delinquent kids. They had been involved in all aspects of Lincoln Hall and did have keen insights into what worked and what didn't. If they started something new, it was sure to work. Bob Wagner could sell the Brooklyn Bridge. He was an idea person. He didn't sleep well and would sit up all night dictating ideas into a tape recorder or he would make a round trip to New York in a day and do the same thing. His ideas were tremendous, but he needed someone around to implement them and see that they worked on a day to day basis... Mike Reis was the complement to Bob's personality. He was purposeful, careful in his decision making and saw to the details. They were a tremendous working combination. Their enthusiasm was contagious. Before word one was on paper about this new project, they had managed to have our whole community of province administrators commit themselves to personally working the new program when it started. I still wonder how they managed to do that. (Maloney, 1986, pp. 113–114)

Br. Robert's powers of persuasion were not limited to the province administrators. He also convinced one of the authors (Grebstein) to design a program of psychological services for the new program and to initially donate his time to providing consulting services (which he has done now for 40 years).

Now that the seeds for a new program had been planted, the issue was how to develop it into a viable program. There was no provision for the placement of delinquents in Rhode Island other than that at the state's training school. The family court judges were forced to send youngsters to the training school with less serious offenses and those who came into foster care as a result of family disintegration due to mental illness, drug and alcohol abuse, and other social problems. The brothers began to develop plans for a residential program with strong ties to the community and the youngsters' families. As Maloney (1986, p. 117) notes:

> The initial program would make use of the Narragansett facility as a residential treatment center. There would be a maximum capacity of thirty residents and these boys would be worked with in groups of ten. Each youngster would participate in an intensive residential experience of counseling, daily living activities and recreational opportunities for approximately nine months to one year. In addition, there would be academic and vocational training in the program's school and each resident and his family could be involved in personal and family counseling. The various components of the program were intended to work closely together toward the aim of returning the youngster to his home more prepared to deal with life in his community.

The long-term plans went beyond the establishment of a residential program and included the creation of smaller group homes in the community that were extensions of the residential program and could serve as transitional placements back to the community, vocational training and apprenticeship programs, and the inclusion of a research component.

One final preliminary step remained: a name change. The original name designated for the new program was the Christian Brothers Youth Center. The brothers recognized that some inaccurate assumptions could result from this name. For example, people might think that only Roman Catholic boys were eligible for treatment. Furthermore, the name might jeopardize the chances of receiving federal grants to help finance the project. In an interview cited by Maloney, Br. Michael Reis describes the brainstorming process that led to the change in the name of the program.

> We were trying to come up with names for weeks. There were all sorts of ideas from the brothers in our community. Some of the names might have been apt, but they could never

> be used! Since we were by the water, words Ocean and Bay were being thrown around. Finally, Brother William Harkins remembered a quote from William Shakespeare. "There is a tide in the affairs of men which, taken at the flood, leads on to fortune, omitted, all the voyage of their lives is bound in shallows and in misery." It was from *Julius Caesar*. We wanted to be that tide in these kids lives! Thus, Ocean Tides. (Maloney, 1986, p. 121)

The process of moving from the developmental stage to the implementation stage encountered formidable obstacles. In addition to the necessity of convincing key political, judicial, and corrections figures of the need and desirability of the program, there were significant practical problems, such as zoning and financial support to solve. Maloney (1986) documents considerable support for the newly designed program from the chief judge of the Family Court, the assistant director of the Department of Corrections, the bishop of Providence, state legislators, the governor, corrections officials, and a variety of other significant people. The biggest hurdle was money. Although the state officials maintained that they wanted the program, they did not want to pay for it. Maloney (1986) described the difficulties the brothers encountered in trying to obtain funding. Ultimately, the brothers obtained partial funding for the program from a federal grant through the 1968 Omnibus Crime Control and Safe Streets Act and through the 1974 Law Enforcement Assistance Act. To obtain the balance of the needed funding, the brothers proposed to take only residents from the training school, thus reducing the cost to the state as a result of the reduced population at the training school. The cost of keeping a youngster at the training school was considerably more than the cost of placing the youngster in the proposed new program, as it still is. For example, in 2013, Ocean Tides was reimbursed by the state at $177.76 per resident per day, which means that it cost the state of Rhode Island approximately $64,882 a year to house one juvenile at Ocean Tides. Compare that to $174,814 a year to house one juvenile at the Rhode Island Training School (Rhode Island Department of Children, Youth, and Families, 2012). Ocean Tides is 63% less expensive to the state than its own youth prison. In the earlier days of the program, a compromise was reached, in which the state raised the amount it was willing to pay and the program lowered its requests. However, the state officials wanted to deduct the amount of money the program had received from the federal grant. They learned that they could have been eligible for receiving a comparable grant had they applied for it. With financial arrangements with the state finally completed on July 15, 1975, the first four boys from the training school were brought to Ocean Tides on August 8, 1975, and the Ocean Tides program began.

CONCLUSIONS

This chapter chronicles major events and changes in juvenile justice in the United States from the 1950s through the establishment of the Ocean Tides program in 1975. The discussion chronicles the events and policies both nationally and locally that shaped and characterized how juvenile delinquents were conceptualized and treated. The authors describe the specific events in Rhode Island that led to the founding of Ocean Tides, and some of the obstacles confronted by the program's developers.

REFERENCES

Battersby, W. J. (1970). *Brother Barnabas: Pioneer in modern social science.* Winona, MN: St. Mary's College Press.

Carkhuff, R. R. (1974). *Cry twice.* Amherst, MA: Human Resource Development Press.

Cohen, L. E., & Land, K. C. (1987). Age structure and crime: Symmetry versus asymmetry and the projection of crime rates through the 1990s. *American Sociological Review, 52,* 170–183.

Crepeau, H. J. (1941). *Rhode Island: A history of child welfare planning.* Washington, DC: Catholic University of America Press.

Dohrn, B. (2002). The school, the child, and the court. In M. Rosenheim, F. E. Zimring, D. S. Tenenhaus, & B. Dohrn (Eds.), *A century of juvenile justice* (pp. 267–309). Chicago, IL: University of Chicago Press.

Field, E. (Ed.). (1902). *State of Rhode Island and Providence plantations at the end of the century: A history.* Boston, MA: Mason.

Gabriel, A. (1948). *The Christian Brothers in the United States: 1848–1948.* New York, NY: Declan X. McMullen.

Handler, J. F., & Zatz, J. (Eds.). (1982). *Neither angels nor thieves: Studies in deinstitutionalization of status offenders.* Washington, DC: National Academy Press.

Lindner, C., & Wagner, R. (1983). The Ocean Tides experiment: Treatment of serious juvenile offenders in an open residential setting. *Federal Probation, 47*(1), 26–32.

Maloney, D. J. (1986). *The Ocean Tides residential, educational and family services program: An organization history 1975–1985* (unpublished doctoral dissertation). Chestnut Hill, MA: Boston College.

Mennel, R. M. (1973). *Thorns and thistles: Juvenile delinquents in the United States, 1825–1940*. Hanover, NH: University Press of New England.

President's Commission on Law Enforcement and Administration of Justice. (1967). *The challenge of crime in a free society*. Washington, DC: Government Printing Office.

Rhode Island Department of Children, Youth, and Families (2012, March). *FY 2012 revised and FY 2013 operating budgets FY 2013–FY 2017 capital budget*. Staff presentation. Retrieved from http://webserver.rilin.state.ri.us/HouseFinance/DCYF%20FY%202013%20Gov%20%28Corrected%29.pdf

Sagi, P. C., & Wellford, C. F. (1968). Age composition and patterns of change in criminal statistics. *The Journal of Criminal Law, Criminology and Police Science, 59*(1), 29–36.

Sanders, W. B. (1970). *Juvenile offenders for a thousand years: Selected readings from Anglo-Saxon times to 1900*. Chapel Hill, NC: University of North Carolina Press.

Shoemaker, D. J. (2009). *Juvenile delinquency*. Lanham, MD: Rowman & Littlefield.

Steffensmeier, D., & Harer, M. D. (1987). Is the crime rate really falling? *Journal of Research in Crime and Delinquency, 24*, 23–48.

Tanenhaus, D. S. (2002). The evolution of juvenile courts in the early twentieth century: Beyond the myth of the immaculate construction. In M. K. Rosenheim, F. E. Zimring, D. S. Tanenhaus, & B. Dohrn (Eds.), *A century of juvenile justice* (pp. 42–73). Chicago, IL: University of Chicago Press.

CHAPTER 2

Currents: Who the Boys Are

The Ocean Tides program has been in operation for nearly 40 years and no comprehensive description of its population has been published to date. In this chapter, the Ocean Tides database is described and chronological changes in that population are identified.

All of the residents in the Ocean Tides program are court-adjudicated male juvenile delinquents with charges serious enough to have been sentenced to at least probation, and, for the great majority of cases, time to serve in the Rhode Island Training School (RITS) for boys (youth prison). Contrary to many private programs, the residents at Ocean Tides are not selected to avoid difficult youngsters. As Lindner and Wagner (1983) noted in their initial description of the program, an important and distinctive feature of the Ocean Tides program is its admission policies. Because it is a private (i.e., non-governmental) agency, it can establish its own criteria for admission. In the past, private institutions have used such a policy to exclude youngsters perceived as more difficult to manage. By using high or more selective admission criteria, private institutions were more likely to contain dependent and neglected children, status offenders, or juveniles who had committed minor crimes. State training schools or youth prisons, on the other hand, having no choice in the selection process, "became the traditional 'dumping grounds' for those children screened out of the private schools" (Lindner & Wagner, 1983, p. 26).

INTAKE CRITERIA

Only boys between the ages of 13 and 17 years are considered for acceptance into the program. Neither religion nor racial or ethnic backgrounds are in any way factors in determining a boy's eligibility for acceptance into the program. The intake policy is flexible and each youngster who is referred is considered on an individual basis. The primary criterion for acceptance is that the youngster will be able to benefit from the program in the opinion of the intake committee. Acceptance is based on the program's ability to satisfy the rehabilitative goals and needs for the youngster and to generate positive development. The program attempts to be both realistic and honest in terms of the clients it serves. As the program is an "open setting" and not a locked facility, it must be cognizant of its responsibility to the surrounding community. When the program was initially established, specific criteria for rejection included (a) youngsters who had not been adjudicated as delinquent; (b) youngsters involved in serious crimes against the person, such as murder or rape; (c) youngsters suffering from serious emotional disorders and/or who have been diagnosed as psychotic; (d) youngsters who are, de facto, addicted to narcotics; (e) youngsters who have a history of arson; and (f) youngsters who, in the judgment of the Intake Committee, would not be able to benefit from the total program. This original plan was short-lived and these intake criteria were modified early on so that all types of offenders who might benefit from the program are now included in the program. For example, a number of youngsters, who are serious drug users, have been admitted to the program and undergo drug testing while in residence. Likewise, data for the present study include all of the residents of Ocean Tides from 1975 to 2007 and show that 14 of the Ocean Tides boys (0.9%) were charged with attempted murder, 68 (4.3%) with arson, 25 (1.6%) with sexual assault against someone younger than 16 years, and 2 (0.1%) with sexual assault of a person between 16 and 18 years of age.

THE OCEAN TIDES DATA PROJECT

The Ocean Tides Data Project is the title given to the task of designing and constructing a massive database that contains information about the boys who resided there since the program's inception in 1975. The authors conducted this research from 2002 through 2012.

When each boy enters the Ocean Tides program, a hard-copy file is compiled, which contains a plethora of information about him and his family. The file folder is numbered and once the boy completes the program, it is archived at the facility. Electronic copies of this information do not exist.

On very modest funding, the authors spent the first year of the project defining terms and creating systematic mechanisms for quantifying the information contained within the files. They created a detailed codebook consisting of 1,930 variables and began to code the data in the files and create the electronic database. Within the first year of data collection, they realized that the tasks at hand were far too time-consuming to complete without assistance. Each boy's folder contained between 150 and 300 pages and took approximately 3 hours to enter. The authors hired and supervised undergraduate students, each of whom worked for one semester earning college credit for the work. Later, they hired a few graduate students and, in 2007, they were granted modest funding to pay students for their work. This enabled them to keep a student on the project for multiple semesters, which saved training time. Data were collected from 2002 through 2012, during which time the authors trained and supervised 38 undergraduate and 5 graduate students from the University of Rhode Island to work as research assistants. Ongoing Institutional Review Board (IRB) approval was maintained over the research period, and every research assistant underwent training and was certified for dealing with human subjects prior to participating in the project.

The recording process involved the careful reading of each report in the hard-copy juvenile records. This was an exacting and time-consuming process that involved careful evaluation, cross-checking of information, and constant supervision and feedback. The authors answered questions that arose, recorded data, and systematically checked students' data entry and their assessment of the information in the folders. This work was conducted inside the Ocean Tides facility because the files themselves could not be taken from the premises for reasons of confidentiality. Data validity was maintained by avoiding any speculation about missing information. The researchers were most vigilant regarding the restriction of speculation. It helped to include an open-ended variable at the end of the database where research assistants could state their opinions, assumptions, and add information that they thought was pertinent but that could not be captured by the existing variables in the database.

Database Size

The resulting Ocean Tides database contains 1,585 cases of boys who entered the program from 1975 through 2006. All analyses in this study include the entire database and no samples unless otherwise noted. Most of the analyses then include from 80% to 100% of the cases.

Missing Data

Missing data in this database result mainly for two reasons. One is the archival nature of the information. Record keeping evolved over the program's 38 years in existence and the cardboard boxes in which most of the hard-copy files are housed were moved from one room to another within the facility. For regular personnel at the facility, it was also physically difficult to refile information when it was necessary to retrieve it from storage. The second reason for missing data concerns the length of stay for boys and the nature of their release. Some boys elope early, for instance, or are transferred out of state where extended family members live and so very little information is available for these residents.

Data Contents

Each boy's hard-copy file contains demographic information about the juvenile and his family (e.g., ethnicity, race, occupation of parents, socioeconomic status, residence); criminal and substance abuse history of parents or parent surrogates; written clinical psychological evaluations based on individual interviews; progress reports from school, social services, and residential staff; educational and medical history prior to being at Ocean Tides, including discharge summaries if the boy was in a psychiatric hospital; interviews with parents and other family members; court records and results of psychological and educational testing; exit interviews; and progress reports of 3- or 6-month follow-up after completing the program.

Dr. Grebstein is responsible for conducting the psychological evaluation interviews at Ocean Tides. The social services staff provides the individual and family counseling. Summaries of the information from these sessions are included as progress notes in each student's record. The social services counselors meet with the juveniles for individual counseling on a weekly basis and less frequently with the families. Family meetings are typically done in the boy's home, or a convenient meeting place, such as the Providence Campus of the Ocean Tides School or one of the extension houses. In addition to regularly scheduled counseling appointments, counseling sessions occur when a resident requests it, when a staff or faculty member requests it, or as the result of a behavioral transgression. The social services staff conducts the exit interviews with boys who successfully complete the 1-year program.

The Psychological Evaluation Interview

The bulk of information that is contained in the interview reports is self-reported by the juveniles, and it is cross-checked with other sources in the records. The reports from the evaluation interviews and counseling sessions are of primary significance to the research project. Dr. Grebstein was responsible for conducting most of the psychological evaluation interviews with the Ocean Tides' juveniles since the program's inception. He developed a systematic routine for conducting the interviews at the program's opening and modified it as the program developed. He follows the same format for every session and records his own summary of information after each session. He then transcribes his notes into a formal written report that is placed in the boy's file.

Each psychological evaluation interview contains the following information: age; ethnicity; a description of the juvenile's behavior, body language, and expressions during the interview; the juvenile's assessment and description of exposure to family violence; psychiatric history; medical history; physical health problems; information about the juvenile's family members, which includes illegal drug and alcohol history; family socioeconomic status (SES) or history; relationships with family members; gang involvement; weapons use; educational history and attitudes about school and education; behavior in school; the most current charges against the juvenile and his placement history; the juvenile's feelings about the offenses he has committed and his current situation; experience with substance abuse; plans for the future; anger management; hobbies, career goals, goals to achieve while residing at Ocean Tides; Dr. Grebstein's perception of the juvenile's personality characteristics; and his clinical (*DSM*) diagnoses and recommendations for treatment (a much more detailed description of Dr. Grebstein's interview style, purposes, and his philosophy on interviewing juvenile delinquents is provided in Chapter 8). The *DSM* is the *Diagnostic and Statistical Manual of Mental Disorders,* which has been developed by and published by the American Psychiatric Association. Data collection for this project was conducted between 2002 and 2012. The information in the boys' files from which the database was constructed came from 1975–2007. The *DSM-I* was published in 1952; *DSM-II* in 1968; *DSM-III* in 1980; *DSM-III-R* (a significantly revised edition) in 1987; *DSM-IV* in 1994; and the *DSM-5* not until 2013. The *DSM* is the standard nomenclature used in the United States by mental health professions to diagnose disorders.

It is important to note that most of the boys perceive their placement at Ocean Tides as a privilege. They see their placement as a second chance, and the accommodations are much more pleasant and less restrictive than youth prison. They are typically cooperative with Dr. Grebstein, and a measurement of cooperation is included in the data. In the years included in the database, only one resident refused to participate in the evaluation conducted by Dr. Grebstein. He was returned to the training school within a week for noncompliance with the program.

The Parent Interview

Parent interviews are conducted with the primary custodial parent and are conducted by the social worker assigned to each boy. The following information is contained within reports from these interviews: family structure and changes over the boy's lifetime; deaths and illnesses of family members; residential mobility; medical and clinical histories of the parents, the juvenile, and his siblings; first-generation family violence; parental assessment of the child's exposure to family violence; criminal history of family members, including the juvenile; juvenile involvement in deviance undetected by legal functionaries; parental abandonment; disciplinary practices; quality of the relationship with the juvenile; the boy's history of behavior and progress as it relates to his formal education; race; and his developmental progress.

Clinical Reports and Testing Results

Clinical reports from agencies other than Ocean Tides are included in the files. Each report bears each boy's age at testing or evaluation, diagnoses (reported following the *DSM-III* to the *DSM-IV*; American Psychiatric

Association, 1994 categorization, and Achenbach scores—these testing procedures are only available in records since the 1980s), and treatment. Many of the juveniles' files contain multiple reports from different years.

Social Services Reports

External contacts with social services are documented in the records, and these files detail the reason for contact. The information that is contained within the social services reports is varied because different people write them, but they do all include the child's age at the time the report was written; the reason for contact with social services; a description of the problem; and the action that was taken by the responding agency. Home assessment reports are included in the majority of the files and include descriptions of the child's neighborhood, home and surrounding area, condition of the living situation, and household crowding.

Educational History and Test Results

A thorough educational history is maintained in the records. Information includes each boy's last school attended and grade level achieved; if dismissed, then a dismissal report is included; the types of schools attended (e.g., private, public); special education status and history, which include educational test scores such as Woodcock Johnson and the Wide Range Achievement Test (WRAT); IQ scores; and overall academic progress.

Court Records

Court records in each boy's file include all contact with juvenile courts. Each court record contains the charged offense; the age of the juvenile at the time of the offense; a description of the transgressions; the juvenile's behavior during the arrest, sentencing, and placement information; and the outcome of each case.

Incident Reports

While juveniles reside at Ocean Tides, staff, teachers, counselors, and social workers are required to write incident reports about the boy's transgressions, and those reports are filed into the juvenile's records.

DESCRIPTION OF OCEAN TIDES BOYS

Ocean Tides is a 1-year program designed to provide early release and skills necessary for success outside the program in legitimate, law-abiding activities. Notably, 62.5% of Ocean Tides boys have graduated from the program. Generally, boys leave Ocean Tides for one of four reasons (see Table A.1 in Appendix A): (a) unauthorized, usually meaning they elope and no follow-up information is in the boy's file (13.1%); (b) they graduate from the program (62.5%); (c) they are returned to the RITS (17.8%); or (d) their stay is otherwise terminated (4%). This final category includes several other reasons. For example, some boys are transferred to another state or country where they have relatives and fall under the jurisdiction of their new residence. A few boys are sent to in-house clinical programs for reasons such as suicidal attempts or serious mental illness, and some boys are transferred to other youth programs outside of the Ocean Tides program and not the RITS.

Age at Entry

Ocean Tides officially accepts boys aged 13 to 17 years, but there have been a few exceptions. For example, two boys entered the program just shy of their 13th birthdays and 17 boys were accepted into the program, probably at one of the local residence houses, past their 18th birthdays. The average age of the Ocean Tides resident, however, is around 16 years. Seventy-eight percent of the boys were from 15 to 17 years of age when they entered the program (n = 1,575, 99.4% response rate). A very small proportion of them are younger than 15 years (12%).

Family or Home SES

SES is broadly defined into five categories that range from lowest to highest (see Table A.2 in Appendix A): (a) the underclass, comprising those who are living in poverty and qualify for substantial government assistance to survive; (b) borderline poverty, which means the family barely scrapes by but does not qualify for welfare assistance; (c) lower middle; (d) middle range; and (e) upper middle economic status. No boys in the study would be considered as affluent. When these families experience delinquency, they often have the resources available to avoid official sanctions. Forty-three percent of the Ocean Tides boys experience some form of extreme poverty. This variable is an assessment of the SES of the boy's family with whom he was residing when he got into the trouble that resulted in his placement at Ocean Tides. Parental employment is one indicator of SES. Only 38% (n = 602) of the boys' biological fathers and 48% (n = 758) of their biological mothers were employed, either full or part time, at the time of the boys' most recent arrest.

Race

Racial identity was obtained for 1,323 of the boys (83.5%; see Table A.3 in Appendix A). Some of the boys' hard-copy files contained their official photographs, such as a copy of a driver's license, a passport, or a photograph taken on entrance into the program. Most of the racial information was obtained from transcripts of parent interviews originally gathered by social workers. Roughly, 47% to 50% of the sample could be considered as racially White. This information covers 31 years, therefore making national or state comparisons is a bit arbitrary. Nonetheless, it is important to note that Rhode Island has always had a disproportionately large White composition. Data from the 2011 U.S. Census indicate that 76.5% of the population in Rhode Island was White non-Hispanic compared to 63.4% nationally for the same year. It also has a relatively low representation of Blacks: 7.2% in Rhode Island in 2011 compared to 13.1% nationally. The Hispanic population is more comparable to national averages primarily due to a large Portuguese population, but is still disproportionate: 12.8% in Rhode Island and 16.7% nationally in 2011.

Race is descriptively important. Individual life experiences are submerged into the culture in which people live. Therefore, others' preconceived ideas about who they are structure those experiences. Biases, such as racism and classism, are ascribed, meaning they are conceived the moment two people see each other and they can overshadow further relations with one another. People often see color or race first and they broadly categorize people by color. For example, while conducting the present research, we discovered that it was common for police officers to record a boy's race in the police reports as either Black or White only, with little, if any attention paid to ethnicity. Hence, non-White Hispanics, Native

Americans, and Black youth were most often recorded on police reports as "Black," while everyone else was recorded as "White." Even Asians were more often recorded as White than they were Asian or non-White. The race variable used in the proceeding analyses is a more traditional categorization in which Hispanic Whites and Whites are coded as (a) White (49.8%); Asians, Blacks, non-White Hispanics, and Native Americans are coded as (b) non-Whites (33.7%; see Table A.4 in Appendix A).

In terms of the racial composition of the data over time, although there were minor fluctuations by year, the non-White population at Ocean Tides rose significantly (Kendall's tau-b = .263, $p = .000$; see Table A.5 in Appendix A). This increase was not limited to a particular racial group, but results are particularly interesting for non-White Hispanics. The first boy in this category arrived at Ocean Tides in 1981, and 65% of all non-White Hispanics arrived from 2000 to 2006, mirroring the overall increase in the U.S. population at large.

Immigration

Boys identified as immigrants in this study are first-generation immigrants, meaning that the boy himself was born in a foreign country. The immigration status was obtained for 91.7% ($n = 1{,}454$) of the sample. Of these boys, 8.3% ($n = 121$) were immigrants (6.62% of the total Ocean Tides population; Table 2.1). Looking at immigration by race provides a closer look, but we do lose 16 cases. Race is missing for these 16 immigrant boys.

The largest category of immigrant boys at Ocean Tides is Hispanic non-White although that group is just more than 2% of the total Ocean Tides population followed by Hispanic White and Puerto Rican, each at less than 1% of the Ocean Tides population.

Family Structure

Family structure refers to the structure of the family with whom the boy was living at the time of his most recent incarceration—the one that resulted in his Ocean Tides residence. Information on who the boy was living with exists for 98% ($n = 1{,}553$) of the sample (see Table A.6 in Appendix A). Among the Ocean Tides boys, about 45% come from single-parent families in one form or another. This is far above national

TABLE 2.1
Immigrant Boys by Race and Ethnicity

RACE	IMMIGRANTS n	PERCENT OF IMMIGRANT POPULATION	PERCENT OF TOTAL OCEAN TIDES POPULATION
Asian	12	10	0.75
Black	7	6	0.44
Cape Verdean	10	9	0.63
Hispanic White	15	13	0.94
Hispanic non-White	37	32	2.33
Hispanic nondescriptive	11	10	0.69
Puerto Rican	15	13	0.94
White	5	4	0.31
All multiracial	3	3	0.18
Totals	*105*	*100*	*6.62*

averages. For comparison, in 1980, 19.5% of U.S. households were single-parent families with children compared to 58.1% of the Ocean Tides population; in 1990, 24% was the national figure compared to 41.9% of Ocean Tides; and in 2000, 27% nationally compared to 46.2% of the Ocean Tides population.

Non-White boys were more likely to live in single-parent households (50.1%) than Whites (43.5%, Kendall's tau-b = −.065, $p = .020$). Furthermore, there is a predictable linear correlation between SES and family structure so that boys in single-parent households were more likely to reside in the lower SESs (Kendall's tau-b = .203, $p = .000$). This is not surprising because it is common knowledge in gender studies that in the event of divorce or separation in the United States, women typically retain primary economic responsibility for their children and their earning potential is about 80% of their male counterparts. Hence, divorce lowers the net worth of women and raises it for men.

Family Stability

Family stability refers to the changing structure of the family unit. Information for this variable exists for 99% ($n = 1{,}569$) of the database (see Table A.7 in Appendix A). "Stable" includes an intact biological family; one biological parent and one long-term stepparent; or a single parent for a minimum of 5 years prior to the boy entering Ocean Tides. Nearly 45% of the sample is from this type of stable family structure. Hence, more than half of the Ocean Tides boys are from unstable to moderately stable (i.e., commonly changing structurally) households.

Parental Drug and Alcohol Abuse

Many of the boys come from homes in which one or more of their parental figures abuses drugs and/or alcohol. Alcohol abuse is more common than serious drug abuse. It is most important to note that 20.8% of the boys' fathers drank heavily and 9.2% of their mothers did.

Family Members' Official Criminal Charges

The most significant predictor for childhood delinquency is parental criminal behavior. Nearly 16% of the Ocean Tides boys' biological fathers had incurred official criminal charges in the boys' lifetimes; 12.7% of their biological mothers did; and 5.1% of the boys had other parental figures or adult relatives in official trouble. A full 17% of the boys had a sibling with criminal charges against him or her.

Parental Abandonment and Rejection

Parental abandonment or rejection imposes incredible hardships on children and families. For the purpose of this study, abandonment refers to a parent who relinquishes all contact with the child, excluding cases in which a parent dies. Rejection refers to emotional rejection of the child regardless of whether or not the parent is still part of the child's life and maintains contact with him. Most often, information about rejection came directly from the juvenile via assessment interviews or reports from social workers. More than 37% ($n = 591$) of the Ocean Tides boys were abandoned by their biological fathers and an additional 1.6% ($n = 25$) were emotionally rejected by them although they remained in

TABLE 2.2
Loss in These Boys' Lives

DEATH	*n*	PERCENT
Biological mother	43	2.7
Biological father	98	6.2
Grandmother	98	6.2
Grandfather	77	4.9
Aunt	29	1.8
Uncle	49	3.1
Stepfather	16	1.0
Other father	13	0.8
Stepmother	1	0.1
Other mother	3	0.2
Sibling	45	2.8
Friend	88	5.6

their lives. More than 10% (n = 166) of the boys' mothers physically abandoned them and an additional 1.8% (n = 29) experienced their mothers' emotional rejection.

Not considered in the abandonment and rejection variables is the death of a parent, which is captured in the next variable. Only losses that the boy stated were significant in his life were counted (Table 2.2). Perhaps the most striking loss these boys experienced was the death of a friend. Recall that the average age of these boys is 16 years, but already 5.6% (n = 88) of them knew a friend who had died.

Child Abuse

Sometimes children are better off when their parents are not in their lives. The number of Ocean Tides boys who have experienced some form of abuse in their lifetimes is staggering. Nearly 46% of the boys experienced emotional abuse by their biological fathers and more than 20% by their biological mothers that was serious enough to make it into their Ocean Tides files. Serious physical abuse and sexual abuse are also problematic. Table A.8 in Appendix A details the abuses suffered by the boys by their family members and other nonrelatives who lived with them.

Of course, there are differences between abuse and constructive discipline that ensues in reaction to bad behavior. The corrective use of force is a controversial issue even among experts in child development. Information about the type of punishment these boys were experiencing at home just prior to entering Ocean Tides is available for 71% (n = 1,126) of the boys (see Table A.9 in Appendix A). Only 16.3% (n = 258) of them were receiving what would be considered as a moderate level of punishment for bad behavior. The rest received no, lenient, harsh, or inconsistent punishment.

Official Charges

Several of the Ocean Tides boys had incurred multiple charges at different times in their young lifetimes prior to entering the facility. Information was recorded on all charges for up to five different official encounters with the courts, and 25 boys incurred charges at least five times in their lifetimes with the youngest one receiving his first official charge at 10 years of age. Six of these boys incurred multiple charges against them during their first judicial encounter.

Throughout the study, the "most recent" crimes refer to those that resulted in placement at Ocean Tides and this information is available for 99.4% (n = 1,575) of the boys (see Table A.10 in Appendix A). These boys were officially charged with a total of 3,182 crimes for their most recent encounters with the judicial system. That is an average of about two charges per juvenile for their most recent encounter. The most commonly occurring official charges were for violation of probation (n = 506, almost 16% of all charges) and breaking and entering (n = 444, 13.9%). Most charges were for nonviolent offenses.

In terms of offenders, 36.8% (n = 584) committed violent crimes and 62.6% (n = 992) committed nonviolent crimes for their most recent legal encounters. It is important to note that this does not mean that 36.8% of the boys were violent offenders. We can only say that they had committed a violent offense for which they were placed at Ocean Tides. Some of the boys' most recent charges may have been for nonviolent offenses, but they may have violent offenses in their past or their violent behavior was not legally detected. For all crimes committed, both recent and past, 830 (52.7%) of the boys were charged with a violent crime at least once in their lifetime, while 745

(47.35%) had been charged with only nonviolent crimes throughout their lifetimes. It is not unusual that overall Ocean Tides houses more violent than nonviolent offenders because juveniles with only nonviolent offenses are often diverted from the justice system or sentenced with home confinement or similar sanctions other than incarceration.

Patterns of Official Charges Over Time

Significant changes are seen over time in the types of charges the boys incurred. Boys entering the program more recently are more likely to have been officially charged with more violent crimes than the boys who entered Ocean Tides in the past (Pearson's $r = .295$, $p = .000$). Specifically, more nonviolent than violent offenders entered the program every year from 1975 through 1990. Beginning in 1991, the pattern changed. From 1991 through 2006 (the most recent year of entry in the database), more violent than nonviolent offenders entered the program each year. To discern whether a consistent pattern of increased violence occurred over time, Pearson's correlations were calculated for the two periods (1975–1990 and 1991–2006). For 1975 to 1990, the correlation was .121 ($p = .003$), indicating that the boys' offenses were becoming more violent across this time period. This was not the case for 1991 to 2006 (Pearson's $r = -.19$, $p = .551$), which means that the ratio of violent to nonviolent charges stabilized after 1991. The general trend found at Ocean Tides is similar to larger national patterns of juvenile arrests. The Office of Juvenile Justice and Delinquency Prevention (OJJDP) identified a slow, but steady, increase in violent charges against juveniles aged 10 to 17 years, beginning around 1988 and peaking at an all-time high in 1994, when it steadily dropped through 2004 (OJJDP).

Race and Official Charges

Non-Whites were more likely to have been arrested for violent than nonviolent offenses (violent = 64.2% and nonviolent = 35.8%). Whites were more likely arrested for nonviolent than violent offenses (violent = 48.2%, nonviolent = 51.8%). This trend is also consistent with OJJDP estimates for national trends.

SES and Official Charges

The relationship between SES and violence is not significant among the Ocean Tides residents (Kendall's tau-b = –.021, p = .290), so there are no discernable differences in violence arrests by SES.

Drug-Related Charges

There were 336 boys (21.2%) charged with drug-related offenses at some point in their lifetimes. There is no correlation between drug-related charges and SES (Kendall's tau-b = –.13, p = .585). Non-Whites were more likely to be charged with drug-related offenses (58.2%) than Whites (42%; Kendall's tau-b = .189, p = .000). Drug-related charges increased over the years (Kendall's tau-b = .172, p = .000) with 62% of all drug charges occurring over the 9 years between 1997 and 2006.

One of the strengths of this database is that it contains information about the boys' general behavior and problem incidents and not just official charges. This information comes from reports from social workers, clinical counselors, parents, teachers, and other community contacts, as explained earlier in this chapter.

Underage drinking and marijuana use are common in this population of boys, with 54.4% (n = 863) of the boys engaging in light to heavy drinking and 52.7% (n = 836) smoking marijuana, both within the year prior to entering Ocean Tides. Some of the boys also used inhalants (1%, n = 16), heroin (0.2%, n = 3), coke or crack (2.9%, n = 46), Ecstasy (0.6%, n = 9), various pills (1.4%, n = 22), and other hallucinogens (2.9%, n = 46). Of course, some of the boys engaged in multiple forms of drug use, but alcohol and marijuana were the most common.

Whites were more likely to use both alcohol (52.7% of Whites and 36% of non-Whites) and marijuana (55.3% of Whites and 49.1% of non-Whites) than non-Whites were. These differences are statistically significant for alcohol use (Kendall's tau-b = –.165, p = .000) and marijuana use (Kendall's tau-b = –.061, p = .027). These findings are particularly interesting because non-Whites were more likely to be charged with these crimes even though they were less likely to engage in these behaviors than Whites. It appears that the drug-related behavior of non-Whites is more heavily scrutinized than for White juveniles.

There are no statistically significant differences between races in the amount of consumption of each of these drugs. So, for example, boys who drank tended to drink about the same amount regardless of race. SES is unrelated to drug and alcohol use.

Gang and Gun Involvement

Involvement with gangs and the illegal use of guns tend to go hand in hand. In this study, 46.6% of boys who were involved with gangs had also handled guns illegally compared to 17.2% of boys who were not in gangs. Involvement with gangs and guns was only recorded in this study if there was clear certainty of involvement. Just 8.4% (n = 133) of the boys were in gangs, and 19.7% (n = 312) had handled guns illegally.

Race is correlated with both gang and gun involvement. Non-Whites were statistically more likely to be involved with gangs than Whites (13.9% of non-Whites and 5.8% of Whites; Kendall's tau-b = .137, $p = .000$), and more likely to handle guns (25.5% of non-Whites and 18% of Whites; Kendall's tau-b = .090, $p = .001$). These findings are consistent with national trends.

Gang involvement was more common for boys in the lower SESs (Kendall's tau-b = −.058, $p = .009$), but illegal gun use was not statistically different by SES (Kendall's tau-b = .025, $p = .257$).

Other Problem Behaviors and Attitudes

Perhaps the richest set of variables in this study measures behaviors and attitudes both prior to entering Ocean Tides and again while they were in residence at the facility (Table 2.3). We focus here on these boys' behaviors and attitudes in the year prior to entering the facility. A "slight" problem means that the boy experienced at least one or two serious incidents. This information offers a unique glimpse into how these boys think and behave.

Some of the more commonly occurring problems include stealing (82.8% of the boys had at least a slight problem with stealing), poor judgment (70.9%), aggression (66.2%), impulsivity (61.1%), truancy (58.9%), and violence (57.7%). It is important to note that some problems one might expect in this population are not highly represented, such as bullying (just more than 9% of the boys). Interestingly, a full 5% of the boys who had behaved violently in their lifetimes were never

TABLE 2.3
Behaviors and Attitudes Prior to Entering Ocean Tides

BEHAVIORS/ATTITUDES	PROBLEM			TOTALS
	Slight	Moderate	Severe	
Aggression	33 (2.1)	194 (12.2)	822 (51.9)	1,049 (66.2)
Antagonistic[a]	58 (3.7)	305 (19.2)	203 (12.8)	566 (35.7)
Attention/ concentration	58 (3.7)	300 (18.9)	239 (15.1)	597 (37.7)
Bullying	27 (1.7)	74 (4.7)	45 (2.8)	146 (9.2)
Emotionally labile	29 (1.8)	116 (7.3)	56 (3.5)	201 (12.7)
Enuresis	16 (1.0)	30 (1.9)	17 (1.1)	63 (4.0)
Entitlement	19 (1.2)	88 (5.6)	35 (2.2)	142 (9.0)
Fights with peers	109 (6.9)	293 (18.5)	156 (9.8)	556 (35.2)
Fire setting	63 (4.0)	43 (2.7)	88 (5.6)	194 (12.2)
Immaturity	60 (3.8)	383 (24.2)	202 (12.7)	645 (40.7)
Impulsive	65 (4.1)	436 (27.5)	467 (29.5)	968 (61.1)
Manipulative	48 (3.0)	195 (12.3)	129 (8.1)	372 (23.5)
Temper	50 (3.2)	309 (19.5)	271 (17.1)	630 (39.7)
Poor judgment	105 (6.6)	432 (27.3)	587 (37.0)	1,124 (70.9)
Problems with authority	67 (4.2)	427 (26.9)	275 (17.4)	769 (48.5)
Risk taking	96 (6.1)	264 (16.7)	274 (17.3)	634 (40.0)
Runaway	86 (5.4)	146 (9.2)	174 (11)	406 (25.6)
Self-centered	31 (2.0)	150 (9.5)	46 (2.9)	227 (14.3)
Stealing	19 (1.2)	44 (2.8)	1,250 (78.9)	1,313 (82.8)
Truancy	59 (3.7)	284 (17.9)	590 (37.2)	933 (58.9)
General violence	56 (3.5)	116 (7.3)	743 (46.9)	915 (57.7)

Note: Percents in parentheses.
[a]Swearing/disrespect.

officially charged with any violent crimes. Hence, if this study relied on official arrest records to identify violent behavior, it would have miscategorized 5% of the boys.

Another problem behavior that is often associated with delinquency, specifically violence, is abuse against animals. Children as young as 2 to 3 years old abused animals at least one time that was significant enough to report in their Ocean Tides files. Some incidents, though abusive, did not result in permanent physical damage to the animal (21 boys, 1.3% of the Ocean Tides population), but 26 boys (1.6%) abused animals inflicting serious damage or death.

Psychological Characteristics

Just 13.9% ($n = 221$) of the boys had ever been referred to a mental health facility; most for less than 1 week. About half of them were referred for assessment only ($n = 106$), and the others for both assessment and treatment.

Only about a quarter of the boys (31.2%, $n = 494$) had been clinically evaluated at any point prior to entering the facility. This makes it impossible to rely on these variables to explore their association with other behaviors. Dr. Grebstein personally interviewed and diagnosed 42% ($n = 669$) of the Ocean Tides boys once they entered the facility. Combined, just 54% ($n = 861$) of the boys received at least one *DSM* diagnosis either at Ocean Tides or prior to their arrival. It is reasonable to assume that only the most severe problems were diagnosed then using these clinical methods.

Three fairly common *DSM* groups of disorders have been associated with delinquency in the research. They are attention deficit hyperactivity disorder (ADHD), conduct disorders, and mood disorders. The ADHD category includes predominantly inattentive type, predominantly hyperactive-impulsive type, combined type, and types not otherwise specified (NOS). Recall that impulsive behavioral assessments reported earlier in this manuscript were as high as 61.1% based on all of the information in the boys' files and including nearly all of the cases in this study, but clinical diagnoses of ADHD-related problems among this limited population were relatively low at 16.5% of the boys ($n = 279$). Hence, if this study relied only on clinical diagnoses of ADHD symptoms, it would have miscategorized 44.6% of the boys.

On the one hand, anyone could argue that all of the Ocean Tides boys have some form of conduct disorder or they would not be there; however, clinical diagnosis for conduct disorder, oppositional defiant disorder, disruptive behavior disorder, and conduct NOS is 54.3% ($n = 861$).

Mood disorders diagnosed among the Ocean Tides boys include depressive and bipolar disorders. Just 12.5% ($n = 198$) of the boys were clinically diagnosed at some point in their young lives with one of these problems. Suicidal tendencies are often associated with depressive disorders. The current study measured three types—suicidal ideation, gestures, and attempts—while residing at Ocean Tides, within 1 year prior to entering the facility, and at any point before that. Suicidal ideation refers to having thoughts about taking one's life, including having a specific plan. Suicidal gestures refer to nonlethal attempts that represent a "cry for help" and do not have the intention of resulting in death. Examples are superficially cutting one's wrists or a mild overdose of medication. Suicide attempts are more serious behaviors that represent genuine attempts to kill one self. Less than 9% (n = 140) of the boys experienced suicidal ideation at some point in their lives, 4.3% (n = 68) of the boys had expressed suicidal gestures, and 2.8% (n = 45) of the boys had attempted suicide. For all three types, the boys were much more likely to have experienced it before 1 year prior to entering Ocean Tides. Seven boys (0.4%) in 31 years had attempted suicide while they were residing at Ocean Tides.

Behavioral Medications

Sometimes the clinical diagnosis of a psychological disorder results in the prescription of behavioral medications. The most widely prescribed behavioral medication at Ocean Tides is antidepressants and then only 2.6% of that population is prescribed these medications (see Table A.11 in Appendix A). Only five (0.3%) boys were prescribed stimulants at Ocean Tides.

Several reasons explain the low prescription rate in this population. First, when boys enter the correctional system in Rhode Island, they are taken off of all psychotropic medications; so few, if any, take these medications when they enter Ocean Tides even if they had previously been prescribed them. Second, it often happens that once a boy is taken out of the disruptive environments they lived in prior to going to Ocean Tides they no longer need these medications. Third, many of these boys come from low-income families that cannot afford psychiatric care and so their disorders may go unrecognized. This is certainly the case for the prescription of stimulants prior to residing at Ocean Tides (see Table A.12 in Appendix A). Remember that this study predates national health care in the United States. Boys with the lowest SES are least likely to be prescribed stimulants—just 9.1% of that population followed by 14.2% of boys in the middle class and 28.6% of boys in the upper middle class.

School Performance

Half of the boys (50.4%, n = 665) received the individual education plans (IEPs). "In the 2010/2011 school year, Rhode Island was tied with Massachusetts for the highest percentage of public school students with IEPs (18%) compared with 13% in the United States" (Rhode Island Kids Count, 2014a). The Ocean Tides school has 32.4% more children on IEPs than the average for Rhode Island. An IEP is a special program that is designed for students who have been identified through an evaluation as having some form of deficit that impacts educational performance and requires some form of special education. There are 14 categories of deficits that qualify. These include learning disabilities, speech or language impairments, emotional disturbance, traumatic brain injury, other health impairments (e.g., attention deficit hyperactivity disorder, Tourette's syndrome, heart condition), autistic spectrum disorders, intellectually disabled (formerly mental retardation), hearing impairment, visual impairment (including blindness), orthopedic impairment, multiple disabilities disorder, deaf-blindness, and developmental delay. There is a fairly lengthy and detailed procedure involved before a youngster is deemed in need of special education. It begins with a teacher noticing a deficit and having a specialist work with the student in the classroom for 4 to 6 weeks to try and help the student improve. The student's progress is evaluated. If there is no improvement, there is an additional 4 to 6 weeks of help that is provided. If there is no improvement after this second period, a Response to Intervention (RTF) team refers the youngster to special education. When special education gets the referral, they have 10 days to call a meeting of the classroom teacher, special education teacher, parent(s), and maybe the speech and language pathologist and school psychologist. They review all the information from the RTF team and decide whether or not to proceed with a full evaluation. Usually they do. The school has 60 days to complete all of the components that comprise a full evaluation. These include a psychological evaluation, a social history, an education evaluation, and a special education evaluation. The team reviews the results and decides if the student is eligible for special education. If the decision is affirmative, the IEP team has 15 days to develop an individual education program.

Most of the Ocean Tides boys did not perform well in school prior to entering the program (see Table A.13 in Appendix A). Response rates for these variables range from 88.9% to 92.4%. Of the boys for whom we have this information, approximately half performed consistently poorly on academic performance (46.8%, n = 741), motivation (55.8%, n = 885), and behavior in school (50.2%, n = 795) throughout their lifetimes. It is safe to say that if these boys had not gotten into trouble with the law, they still probably would not have completed school successfully.

Poor educational development is often the result of poor physical or emotional childhood development. However, only 7.4% (n = 118) of the boys had developed below average as reported by their medical histories (see Table A.14 in Appendix A). About 28% (n = 309) of the boys experienced chronic physical health problems that ranged from chronic ear infections and asthma to seizure conditions. National- and state-level estimates of child development are unreliable for comparison because only 48% of pediatricians administer child development screenings in the United States and about half of Rhode Island children receive the same kind of testing by health care professionals and special programs (Rhode Island Kids Count, 2014b).

Career Goals and Hobbies

During the interviews with Dr. Grebstein, boys were asked about their career goals and what hobbies they enjoy (Tables A.15 and A.16 in Appendix A). Information for these variables was sometimes also available in other portions of the files from interviews with parents, social workers, or teachers. Overall, relatively few of the boys expressed either having career goals or hobbies. Engaging in various sports was the most popular hobby among these boys, and joining the armed forces was the career goal they most often expressed. Interestingly, some of the boys had career goals in legal professions (2.6%), such as policing. Perhaps there are opportunities to build mentoring relationships through common ground with law enforcement officers.

CONCLUSIONS

In a nutshell, these boys are troubled. More specifically, this population tends to experience life differently from other boys their age in mainstream society. They are more likely to be economically and socially poor, lacking in basic education and social support networks. They have had little if any structure in their daily lives, and, rightly so, have low aspirations for their future success. They come to Ocean Tides incomplete, not whole with important pieces of life's puzzle missing. Likewise, they have often encountered negative experiences that most kids have not. They are not broken because that would imply that in spite of having all of the required pieces, they no longer function correctly. We also cannot assume that they are inherently bad or evil either as too many essential pieces of their lives are missing to make that judgment. It seems befitting of their predicament that any attempts to correct their illegal behavior need to begin by making them whole, filling in the structural and emotional gaps they so desperately need to function legitimately in society.

REFERENCES

American Psychiatric Association. (1994). *Diagnostic and statistical manual of mental disorders* (4th ed., text rev.). Washington, DC: Author.

Lindner, C., & Wagner, R. (1983). The Ocean Tides experiment: Treatment of serious juvenile offenders in an open residential setting. *Federal Probation, 47*(1), 26–32.

Rhode Island Kids Count. (2014a). *Children enrolled in special education.* Retrieved from www.rikidscount.org/matriarch/documents/Ind59.pdf

Rhode Island Kids Count. (2014b). *Young children with developmental delays & disabilities.* Retrieved from http://www.rikidscount.org/Portals/0/Uploads/Documents/YCDDD%20IB%20Full%20Print%281%29.pdf

CHAPTER 3

Explaining the Ocean Tides: Theory

In this book, the authors focus on the juvenile offender and his life prior to encountering the juvenile justice system, contrary to many other approaches that focus on what is wrong with the juvenile justice system and how to fix it. We look here for direction that may inform prevention and rehabilitation strategies, rather than ask how the justice system can be fixed to properly incarcerate and then reintegrate youthful offenders back into society.

In the previous chapter, we identified several positive components of these boys' lives that are missing, and some negative experiences that may lead to deviant behaviors. To understand how all the pieces of their lives fit together, we turn to theories from multiple disciplines that help to explain why some juvenile boys are delinquent and some are not, thus informing rehabilitative programs that can really work.

It is important to understand that most criminals are very similar to noncriminals in most respects and that everyone has the potential, given the right or wrong circumstances, to commit crime. Everyone sits in some place along a continuum that stretches from noncriminal to criminal, and theories identify and explain which experiences and circumstances move someone closer to committing a crime or further away from it. Each person's location on this line is fluid, shifting in one direction or the other ever so slightly throughout the day, week, month, and his or her life. The same experience emits different pressures at different life stages and ages, and experiences interact in ways that can exacerbate movement on this line toward or away from criminal behavior. Not everyone interprets his or her experiences in quite the same

Before getting poor grades	*After getting poor grades*
No Crime ----------Sam---- Crime	No Crime ----------Sam---- Crime
No Crime -----Bob--------- Crime	No Crime --------------Bob--Crime

FIGURE 3.1 Crime likelihoods.

way either; so simply creating a shopping list of pressures to predict criminal behavior is insufficient.

To illustrate this, let us say that Bob begins his week at the halfway point on this continuum between noncriminal and criminal (Figure 3.1), and Sam is a little closer to criminal.

Bob and Sam both perform poorly in school that week, failing one assignment after the next, but Sam just does not care. He has no prospects for continuing his education, and a formal education is just not emphasized in his household; so he remains in the same place on this continuum regardless of his current situation. Bob, on the other hand, plans to go to college; so he internalizes his experience differently than Sam does and starts to think about cheating to improve his grades. Now Bob may be closer to crime than Sam. The opportunity to cheat on an important examination arises, and Bob does it, is caught, and the transgression is documented on his permanent academic record. Although his parents hire a tutor and reassure him that, with a little hard work, he can succeed without cheating, Bob now knows how to cheat. It is also more important now than ever before for Bob to get good grades because of that mark against him on his permanent record. In spite of having admirable goals and the resources necessary to achieve them, Bob continues to cheat, but Sam never does.

In this example, several mechanisms are at play that explain why someone *decides* to commit a crime, or, as in this case, engages in delinquency. Bob clearly has low self-control but that by itself does not explain his behavior. In fact, it is likely that Sam also has low self-control, which may be why he does not care when he fails. By definition, anyone who commits a crime has low self-control, but not everyone who has low self-control will commit a crime. Crime is complex because people are complex. They are the totality of their own life experiences, which include the people in their lives; the places they go to school and places where they live; and their races, ages, genders, socioeconomic statuses, cultural beliefs, norms, values, spiritual beliefs, and personalities. The commission of crime is influenced by all of these aspects, and because everyone's life experiences are somewhat unique, a theory that explains why someone commits a crime has to consider multiple factors and multiple explanations for various ways in which these factors may combine to lead to criminal behavior. Criminological theories that take this approach are called general theories of crime.

Robert Agnew's general theory of crime integrates leading explanations for deviant behavior from strain theory, rational choice, social learning, self-control, social support, biology, psychology, routine activities, social control, labeling, and social disorganization theory (Agnew, 2005). This general theory of crime is cross-disciplinary and addresses risk factors and explanations for crime at the individual, group, community, and cultural levels. The theory has evolved over time and the approach it takes to explain crime and delinquency is at the cutting edge of criminology.

General theories of crime are intended to explain a wide range of criminal behaviors that occur under most circumstances and in all possible contexts. Creating a general theory of crime is a complex task that Gottfredson and Hirschi (1990) undertook following a long tradition of social control theories (Gottfredson & Hirschi, 1990; Hirschi, 1969; Nye, 1958; Reckless, 1961; Reiss, 1951; Toby, 1957). Social control theories assert that restraints on behavior are necessary early in life to curb delinquency, and that, over time, people develop self-control. People who lack these restraints are likely to deviate from normative society. The loci of responsibility in the development of self-control are family, school, and individual personality. After a decade of research, Gottfredson and Hirschi's (1990) general theory of crime is "one of the strongest known correlates of crime" (Pratt & Cullen, 2000, p. 952). However, the theory pays scant attention to other important aspects of social life that contribute to criminal behavior, such as criminal opportunity, community, culture, formal education, peer groups, and work. Researchers actively debate the extent to which Gottfredson and Hirschi's theory is generally applicable and can, by itself, sufficiently explain crime given its limited scope.

Piquero and Tibbets (1996) find that the rational choice theory more effectively explains crime than self-control does. This theory contends that would-be criminals carefully calculate the outcome costs and benefits of committing a crime, and decide by choosing the route in which costs are minimized and benefits are accelerated (Cornish & Clarke, 2006). Hence, these researchers find that criminals do not lack self-control, but have calculated costs and benefits and choose to engage in the behavior that they judge as most beneficial. This process actually involves great self-control. Pratt and Cullen's (2000) thorough meta-analysis of 10 years of research on self-control identifies variables from the social learning theory that more effectively explain criminal behavior than either social control or rational choice does. Criminals may learn how to justify criminal behavior and how to rationalize their choices, which in turn, increases the likelihood of future crime. Hence, it is possible that some aspects of the theories explain primary deviance, but different explanations may be needed to explain subsequent crime.

Akers's (2006) social learning theory blends components of differential association and techniques of neutralization theories. Differential association theories identify how people learn to be delinquents, and techniques of neutralization are learned ways to neutralize potential feelings of guilt for committing a crime. At the core of Akers's (2006) theory is the individual adoption of definitions that are favorable to crime over those that are not through differential associations, differential reinforcements, and imitation. Differential associations refer to direct exposure to criminal others, norms, and values. Greater exposure to crime increases the likelihood that someone will commit another crime, as in Bob's situation in the earlier example. Patterned rewards for criminal behavior exacerbate the situation and reinforce it (Akers, 2006).

Social learning theories successfully predict crime because rather than reducing their explanations for crime to a single factor, they emphasize a process by which some experiences in life may lead to criminal behavior. Criminological theories provide a veritable treasure chest of logical explanations for crime; however, each theory is rather reductionist in its tendency to overemphasize a single explanation or component and exclude all others. Robert Agnew explains the process by which elements from each of these theories lead to crime through efforts to relieve the strain they create. Van Wyk, Benson, and Harris (2000) find that when compared to self-control, the strain theory is more effective in predicting certain types of crime. Strains are events or conditions that are disliked generally by most everyone (objective strains), or just by the individual (subjective strains; Agnew, 2006b). Nobody particularly likes failing assignments in school, but some people like it even less than others. Strains can be experienced vicariously, too; Bob's parents were probably none too happy with his grades; they can be personal; or they can be anticipated, meaning that an individual may worry that a stressful condition or event will occur or continue (Agnew, 2006b).

Strain results from blocked goals (Agnew, 2006a; Merton, 1938). Agnew (2006a) argues that strains influence crime through (a) the prevention of goal attainment, and goals may include money, autonomy, and masculinity for example; (b) the removal of or threat to remove things that are positively valued; and (c) the presentation of or threat of "noxious or negatively valued stimuli" (Agnew, 2006b). In other words, the person perceives an event as bad or unwanted. Some strains that are of "high magnitude" or "are seen as unjust" are more likely to lead to crime than others, especially if they "are associated with low control," and/or "create some pressure or incentive to engage in criminal coping" versus the use of legitimate means (Agnew, 2005, p. 27). People who face strain under these conditions have increased likelihood of committing crime if their behavior is reinforced, they are pressured into crime, or they are motivated to do it (Agnew, 2006b).

Agnew's general strain theory (GST) explains the processes by which some experiences increase the likelihood of criminal behavior. In his groundbreaking 2005 publication *Why Do Criminals Offend?*, he incorporates sources of strain from traditional theories and explains how they influence this process and lead to criminal behavior. In so doing, he creates a single multilevel cross-disciplinary explanation that addresses why criminals offend, and why they commit specific crimes for all types of offenses at different life stages. It is a true general theory of crime. Some of the most unique aspects of this theory are its ability to explain why the vast majority of people who experience strains, like Sam and Bob, never commit serious crimes and it explains why they can age out of crime altogether. This theory then is most useful for explaining juvenile delinquency and holds great potential to inform rehabilitation strategies.

AGNEW'S GENERAL THEORY OF CRIME

Agnew's general theory of crime is layered and the basic components of the theory are couched within each layer. His GST explains the process by which these layers influence crime. Working from the structural level toward the individual, experiences in each subsequent inner layer are affected by the outer ones. The effects of each layer on the next can occur

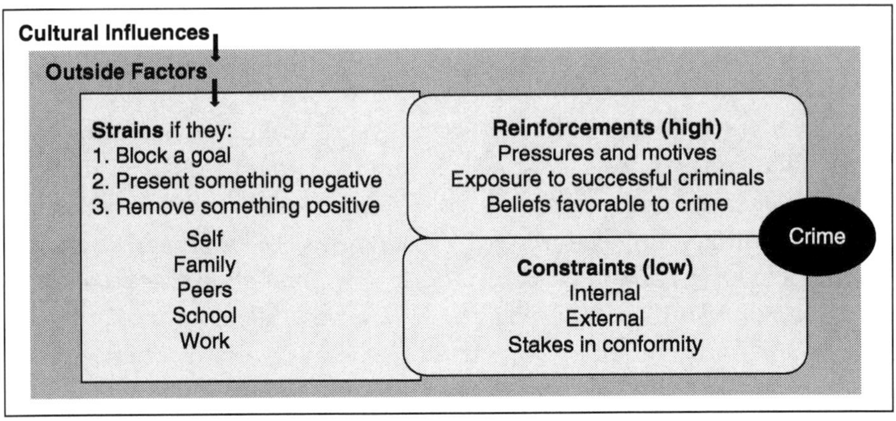

FIGURE 3.2 Agnew's general theory of crime.

simultaneously. He calls these layers starting with the outermost one "culture influences," then there are "outside factors," "life domains," and "constraints" and "reinforcements" (Figure 3.2).

Cultural Influences

Agnew calls the outermost layer of the theory "cultural influences." This is essentially the social structure. Although Agnew does not describe this layer fully in his publications, it is important to understand it in order to recognize the theory's cross-cultural and global reach. From a macro-sociological perspective, the social structure is made up of social institutions that are present in all known societies but they look different between cultures and can change over time within a society. They are patterns of ideas loosely shared within a society that define its main components—the building blocks of a society. People are socialized and guided by these institutions about the roles they play in each of them. They include education, family, religion, medicine, law, government, social control, economy, and labor. People in every known society share some concept of each of these institutions, and these concepts are not concrete, nor stagnant. Take, for example, family. In American society, our concept of family has changed over time and is more inclusive of a diverse array of individuals now than it was in the 1970s. Today we call a single mother and her child a family, whereas in the 1970s, we were more inclined to think of a child living in this arrangement as lacking a family or being in a broken home. No matter how family is defined, imagine a society with no concept of family, and it is not a society. The same is true for the other social institutions.

Social institutions allow societies to function and provide for well-rounded life experiences. They function best when equal importance is established for all social institutions; however, imbalances can occur that create problems for a society. Social institutions are created by values, patterns of ideas in society, but of course everyone does not share the same exact values. Institutions are shaped, then, by those members of a society who have the greatest influence—the greatest amount of social capital—to serve those other members of society whose ideas are similar and to maintain the status quo. If White males have advantages in our social system, then they have the loudest voice and they use it to keep things that way. Social inequalities arise not by mistake but by design, through social policies, formal and informal rules, and laws.

The most crucial imbalance is one that creates mono-institutionalism. This is a situation in which one social institution is awarded greatest prominence and the others suffer. Many social theorists assert this has happened in American culture, and the dominant institution is the economy (see, e.g., Christie, 2004; Messner & Rosenfeld, 2002). In a capitalist society, this means that money dominates all other social institutions and how this society defines them.

In Agnew's theory, these "cultural influences"—the ways in which members of a society define their social institutions—shape relationships and define roles for a culture. Agnew (2005, p. 149) states, "these larger forces...condition the effect of the more immediate outside factors on the life domains." If we want to learn why individuals commit crime, then we have to be cognizant of these cultural influences. We have to recognize that patterns of concentrated low educational attainment, incarceration, or poverty for a particular race or location are socially constructed and, therefore, these situations can be changed.

Outside Factors

"Outside factors," according to Agnew (2005), include biological influences; sociodemographic influences, such as age, sex, race, or ethnicity; and community characteristics. The ways in which a society defines its social institutions and the imbalances among those social institutions in any given society create social inequalities between members of a society based on biological differences and these demographic characteristics. These inequalities mean that people within the society do not each have equal access to social capital, which are the valuable assets within a society. In a capitalist society, social capital might be money or status; in a sexist society, it can be masculinity or simply being male; and in a racist society, it includes the color of one's skin. Social capital is what ultimately determines who wins and who loses in terms of access to success. A society that is mono-institutional and specifically one in which money is power, capital is the most treasured asset and anything that helps to increase wealth is most valuable. It provides advantage. Schwalbe (2008) perhaps explains it best. He identifies characteristics, such as being White and male, as elements of social capital along with the more obvious elements of higher education and money. Even simply having a car to get back and forth to work and certainly having a steady job are all elements of social capital. Agnew (2005) suggests that even biology can be an element of social capital. The structural institutions in a society—the places where our social institutions are played out daily—such as schools, jobs, courts, and even hospitals are designed for fully functioning able-bodied people. People who can walk, think rationally, see, and hear among other things have advantage. Just imagine a child who has attention deficit disorder being asked in the first grade to sit down, be still, be quiet, and pay attention because that is the way we educate people in this society. It becomes very obvious why these children often face difficulties in school.

Imagine a child who is fully functioning physically and emotionally but whose parents lack financial resources. That child will go to a school that is underequipped to prepare him or her for college. He or she will grow up in a neighborhood where other people do not go on to college. The neighborhood may be disorganized and so lack the ability to maintain social control. Inequalities by age, race, ethnicity, gender, socioeconomic status, and biological ability structure experiences in everyday life—in the life domains as Agnew (2005) calls them.

Strains in the Five Life Domains

Agnew (2005) identifies five life domains that are essentially the social places where life happens. They include the self, family, school, peers, and work. Ideally, if everything functions appropriately—the self is stable and adaptive; family is supportive; school educates; peers provide for enjoyable socialization; and work provides our financial, creative, and some emotional needs—then there is no room for crime. Everyone will experience some problems at least at some point in his or her lifetime in at least one of these life domains. Problems are strains that can increase the likelihood of criminal behavior if met with the right reinforcements for crime in the absence of certain constraints against it (Agnew, 2005).

Variables in the five life domains exemplify various types of strain—they prevent goal attainment, remove or threaten to remove things that are positively valued, or they present or threaten to present negatively valued stimuli. For instance, the family domain includes aspects of poor parenting practices, such as negative bonding, poor supervision and discipline, family conflict, child abuse, the absence of positive parenting, and criminal parents and/or siblings (Agnew, 2005). Associations between these experiences and criminal behavior are strong in the theoretical literature from many disciplines, and these associations are strongly supported by empirical evidence. All of the variables in Agnew's theory have been carefully identified based on sound empirical research. Strains that arise in the self-domain are irritability, low self-control, and related problems, such as having a tendency to become easily upset, blaming others for problems, and experiencing intense emotional reactions, chronic anger, low empathy, impulsivity, sensation seeking, and lack of motivation. In the school domain, strains include negative school experiences, such as negative bonding, poor academic performance, little time on homework, low educational and/or occupational goals, poor supervision and/or constructive discipline, negative treatment by teachers, and the absence of positive teaching. The peer life domain includes having close friends who engage in crime, peer conflict and/or abuse, and unstructured or unsupervised time. Finally, strains in the work life domain include unemployment or bad jobs that are characterized by poor supervision and/or constructive discipline at work, negative bonding to work, poor work performance, poor working conditions, and criminal coworkers.

Strains in the life domains are not weighted equally by all people. Remember the earlier example of Bob and Sam. They both performed poorly on schoolwork. The presence of a potential strain-producing experience does not magically lead to crime. If that were true, then everyone would be a criminal. How the experience is interpreted is important. Only if the strain is felt as the presentation of something negative, removes something positive, or blocks a goal, will it actually increase the likelihood of crime. People who experience strains seek relief from them, and although there are several ways to relieve strain, people have differential access to legitimate, law-abiding ways to do it. Relief is dependent on social capital. Sometimes crime provides such relief, albeit a temporary relief. Criminal coping is relatively easy but it can present additional strains; so the decision to commit a crime is tempered by constraints and reinforcements.

Constraints and Reinforcements

At any given time, both constraints against crime and reinforcements for it are at play, tugging slightly in one direction or the other. Constraints can be internal, external, or come in the form of stakes in conformity (Agnew, 2005). Internal constraints may be the likelihood that others will detect and sanction an individual's crime, concern over such sanctions, an individual's own moral reaction to his or her crime, and satisfaction with his or her conventional pursuits. External constraints include laws and rules and the people who enforce them whether they are parents or police. Stakes in conformity are things and people who are important to you and that you fear you would lose if you committed a crime. They can include the attachment or respect from significant others, a good job, an impending educational degree, or even maintaining a good reputation or social status. Constraints can prevent someone from choosing to cope with strain by engaging in criminal activities.

Reinforcements, on the one hand, encourage criminal coping. They include pressures and motives, exposure to successful criminals, and beliefs that are favorable to crime (Agnew, 2005). Pressures and motives are not the same things, but the same event can exert both a pressure and a motive at the same time. Pressures push toward criminal coping, whereas motives pull or entice. Think of pressures as almost being out of one's own control. Bob saw no other alternative than cheating on his examination and, therefore, felt that he had no choice but to do it. The reward or motive was to obtain a good grade.

Exposure to successful criminals is one of the strongest crime predictors. Criminals learn the tricks of the trade from one another and obtain the tools of the trade. Increased exposure to other criminals normalizes not only these behaviors but also criminal beliefs that reinforce criminal learning. Sykes and Matza (1957) explain that criminals learn ways to neutralize guilt they might feel by committing a crime. Believing that a victim had it coming or that a law against something is just ridiculous neutralizes guilt and reinforces criminal decision making.

CONCLUSIONS

Agnew's general theory of crime culls decades of empirical evidence from research and explanations for crime and delinquency from multiple theories and disciplines that identify experiences that lead to crime and explain the processes that connect them with criminal outcomes. Crime is a way of coping with strains that come from cultural, social, and individual mechanisms in the imbalance of reinforcements over constraints against criminal coping. Multiple layers of explanation translate into multiple areas of intervention in the prevention of criminal behavior. For those who are already engaged in crime, like the Ocean Tides boys, this theory can guide rehabilitation efforts.

REFERENCES

Agnew, R. (2005). *Why do criminals offend? A general theory of crime and delinquency.* Los Angeles, CA: Roxbury.

Agnew, R. (2006a). General strain theory: Current status and directions for further research. In F. T. Cullen, J. P. Wright, & M. Coleman (Eds.), *Taking stock: The status of criminology theory, advances in criminology theory.* New Brunswick, NJ: Transaction.

Agnew, R. (2006b). *Pressured into crime: An overview of general strain theory.* Los Angeles, CA: Roxbury.

Akers, R. (2006). A social learning theory of crime. In F. T. Cullen & R. Agnew (Eds.), *Criminological theory: Past to present: Essential readings* (3rd ed., pp. 134–146). Los Angeles, CA: Roxbury.

Christie, N. (2004). *A suitable amount of crime.* London, UK: Routledge.

Cornish, D. B., & Clark, R. V. (2006). Crime as a rational choice. In F. T. Cullen & R. Agnew (Eds.), *Criminological theory: Past to present: Essential readings* (3rd ed., pp. 421–426). Los Angeles, CA: Roxbury.

Gottfredson, M., & Hirschi, T. (1990). *A general theory of crime.* Stanford, CA: Stanford University Press.

Hirschi, T. (1969). *Causes of delinquency*. Berkeley, CA: University of California Press.

Merton, R. (1938). Social structure and anomie. *American Sociological Review, 3,* 672–682.

Messner, S., & Rosenfeld, R. (2002). *Crime and the American dream* (2nd ed.). Belmont, CA: Wadsworth.

Nye, F. I. (1958). *Family relationships and delinquent behavior*. New York, NY: John Wiley.

Piquero, A., & Tibbetts, S. G. (1996). Specifying the direct and indirect effects of low self-control and situational factors in offenders' decision making: Toward a more complete model of rational offending. *Justice Quarterly, 13*(3), 481–510.

Pratt, T. C., & Cullen, F. T. (2000). The empirical status of Gottfredson and Hirschi's general theory of crime: A meta-analysis. *Criminology, 38*(3), 931–964.

Reckless, W. (1961). A new theory of delinquency and crime. *Federal Probation, 25,* 42–46.

Reiss, A. J. (1951). Delinquency as the failure of personal and social control. *American Sociological Review, 16,* 196–207.

Schwalbe, M. (2008). *The sociologically examined life: Pieces of the conversation* (3rd ed.). Boston, MA: McGraw-Hill.

Sykes, G. M., & Matza, D. (1957). Techniques of neutralization: A theory of delinquency. *American Sociological Review, 22*(6), 664–670.

Toby, J. (1957). Social disorganization and stake in conformity. *Journal Criminal Law and Criminology, 48,* 12–17.

Van Wyk, J. A., Benson, M. L., & Harris, D. K. (2000). A test of strain and self-control theories: Occupational crime in nursing homes. *Journal of Crime and Justice, 23*(2), 27–44.

CHAPTER 4

An Undertow: Personal Child Abuse Victimization and Exposure to Parental Interpersonal Violence

In his general theory of crime, Agnew (2005) explains that family is the most influential of the five life domains because it is where people develop the characteristics of the self that then affect every other aspect of life at every life stage and in all contexts. Family is also the most prominent life domain in childhood, although its effects wane in adolescence; so it is a good place to look for potential causes for delinquent behaviors that occur later in life.

The strain theory identifies the presentation of "noxious stimuli" as a major source of strain (Agnew, 2005). For children, that strain can be poor parenting. Some of the worst sources of strain that children experience occur in the home as personal abuses. The negative effects of emotional, physical, and sexual abuse against children are so well documented that they are considered as common knowledge even outside of research communities. Thousands of studies have been conducted from many different perspectives and the overall consensus is that child abuse causes serious short-term and long-term problems. This body of research, though, is not free of problems. It suffers to some extent from the difficult nature of studying such a sensitive and often private issue that affects a population that is, ironically, generally protected from researchers. Nonetheless, at least the direct physical, sexual, and emotional assaults children experience are well studied overall. However, one type of child abuse—parental interpersonal violence (PIPV)—has gained attention from researchers over only the past few decades; so much less is understood about it.

Domestic violence among adults occurs with children present in the home in as much as 48% of families that seek clinical mental health assistance (McDonald, Jouriles, Norwood, Ware, & Ezell, 2000). These acts of violence are not isolated events in these families; on average they occur once or twice per year (McDonald et al., 2000). Hamby, Finkelhor, Turner, and Ormrod (2011) have conducted the most comprehensive nationally representative study to date on exposure to PIPV. Data gathered from 4,549 respondents in 2008 revealed that 6.6% of American youth were exposed to PIPV within the past year, whereas national lifetime estimates are as high has 26%, with 90% of victims actually witnessing physical abuse between parents firsthand (Hamby et al., 2011). Lewis, Siegel, and Lewis (1984) reported that fifth- and sixth-grade children rated parental conflict as one of their top three most stressful life events.

People would generally agree that children who are physically or sexually abused should be separated from the abusing member of the family. This is done for two reasons: (a) to stop the abuse and (b) to begin the physical and emotional healing process. However, courts still typically try to keep children with their families if they are being exposed to PIPV. The guiding philosophy of the courts is that this type of abuse is just not as damaging to children as removing them from the home might be, even though evidence is mounting to suggest otherwise. Removing children from these destructive environments may reduce their ill effects and not only help the children who are experiencing the exposure, but also contribute to curbing delinquency that may result from it. This is a particularly significant issue for court-adjudicated children. If a child gets into legal trouble, he or she may be placed on home confinement, and if that child is exposed to PIPV in the home, then it may exacerbate the trouble instead of curbing it.

Most of what is known about the long-term effects of exposure to PIPV suggests that they linger on into adolescence and adulthood; hence, although removing children from abusive situations may prevent further damage, the emotional and other ill effects may not be reversible. Studies find strong correlations between past violent victimization and exposure to PIPV and future violent behavior, but these studies do not provide a complete picture because they rely on adult respondents recalling traumatic childhood events. Longitudinal or other methods that measure violent behavior before and after removing the child from the abusive context are rare and where they do exist, they are based on samples that are too small for statistical analysis. The Ocean Tides data provide a great opportunity for a more thorough analysis of the effects of direct child abuse and exposure to PIPV on delinquent males.

The 1990s probably produced the greatest number of publications to date on the effects of childhood exposure to PIPV. A comprehensive review of the literature was conducted by Onyskiw in 2003. She reviewed 47 studies published over two decades. She found that, in general, exposure to PIPV increases the incidence of physical health problems, obsessive-compulsive disorders, posttraumatic stress disorder (PTSD), attention problems, anxiety, depression, aggression, self-blame, nervousness; and decreases are found in developmental milestones, academic performance, self-concept, and social competence or functioning. Boys tend to experience more externalizing behavioral problems, such as conduct disorder, whereas girls tend to internalize the effects as self-blame or self-abuse. Peer aggression and bullying result from exposure to family violence as do antisocial behavior, violent crime, substance abuse, further delinquency, and adult criminality (Baldry, 2003; Edleson, 1999; Osofsky, 1999). Age-related outcomes are indicated in a few studies, which reveal that older children have often experienced greater exposure to PIPV simply because they have had more time to accumulate these experiences. Cuevas, Finkelhor, Shattuck, Turner, and Hamby (2013) conducted some of the only analysis that examines the relative ill effects of exposure to PIPV between demographic groups. They found little differences to indicate who is more likely to be exposed to PIPV by socioeconomic status (SES), ethnicity, family structure, disability status, school performance, or physical features (Cuevas et al., 2013). It appears that exposure to PIPV is an equal-opportunity offense against children and adolescents, much in the same way as other abuses against children.

Most research on co-occurrence or polyvictimization indicates that children who are personally abused are often also exposed to PIPV (O'Keefe, 1994), and the ill effects of personal child abuse increase in the presence of exposure to PIPV (for a review, see Onyskiw, 2003). On average, studies using clinical samples find that about 40% of personal child abuse victims are also exposed to PIPV (Onyskiw, 2003). Some research studies indicate that the level, or seriousness, of exposure to PIPV increases the ill effects (Jaffe, Wolfe, Wilson, & Zak, 1986; Jouriles et al., 1998). It is important then to examine the effects of personal abuses and exposure to PIPV in the same sample.

PERSONAL CHILD ABUSE, EXPOSURE TO PIPV, AND VIOLENT BEHAVIOR

Most studies on the effects of exposure to PIPV and on personal child abuse do not isolate violent outcomes from more general aggression. Aggression is broadly defined in the literature as anything from having bad thoughts about someone to physically injuring them. The few studies that do focus on physically violent outcomes typically spotlight adult interpersonal violence (see, e.g., Murrell, Merwin, Christoff, & Henning, 2005). Stith et al. (2000) conducted a meta-analysis of 39 studies either published or otherwise professionally presented between 1978 and 1997 and found weak to moderate effects of exposure to PIPV on this type of violent behavior. Ehrensaft et al. (2003) examined 543 cases over 20 years ending in 1983 and found that child physical abuse increases adult violent offending, although they did not assess exposure to PIPV or gender differences in their sample.

Wekerle and Wolfe (1999) studied 1,317 high school students from 10 high schools and found that the best predictor of adolescent male violence against female partners is exposure to violence at home. Steinberg (2000) conducted a longitudinal study examining pathways to delinquency and found similar results. It is generally accepted among researchers that children who are exposed to PIPV experience emotional and behavioral problems that can reach into adulthood and that these experiences often lead to violent behaviors, but the number of studies that directly test this assumption is very low and empirical results are inconclusive.

Samples of Youth Exposure to PIPV

Studies on child victims of abuse are difficult to conduct. National organizations tally statistics on reported abuse, but experts estimate that those numbers dwarf in comparison to the number of children who experience abuses that are undetected by authorities. Academic and other researchers continue to develop innovative methodological approaches and to employ sampling procedures that may increase discovery, but the private nature of families in general combined with intense public disapproval of child victimization inhibits child abuse disclosure. Child sources of information about their own abuse are tricky, too, because they may not understand their experiences or be able to articulate them well to adults. Exposure to PIPV is difficult to ferret out as well, especially because most information about children is gathered directly from those who may be exposing their children to the abuse. Few parents would admit to fighting in front of their children.

One sampling problem identified in the research is relying on a single source of information about children exposed to PIPV (Holden, 2003). Often the source is the mother, and that is problematic because she is typically experiencing direct trauma from the abuse, so her recollection and interpretation of the events may not be reliable (Appel & Holden, 1998). Children whose parents are separated or divorced may be exposed to PIPV in either household (or both) and one parent may not be aware of the events that occur in the other household.

Holt, Buckley, and Whelan (2008) reviewed the literature on children exposed to PIPV and identified several sampling shortcomings in this body of work. From 1995 through 2000, most of these studies used either very small clinical samples or generated samples from women's shelters. Some researchers worried that samples from women's shelters might overrepresent people from lower SES (Kerig, 1998). It also seems reasonable to assume that without a national health care system in place, studies that focus exclusively on clinical samples might overrepresent wealthier people who can afford to seek psychological and psychiatric assistance. Whether they exaggerate or ignore the experiences of specific economic classes, clinical and shelter samples do not produce reliable results about the general population.

National samples seem to be the gold standard in social research, but research on children presents special problems. The only nationally representative study of youth exposed to PIPV uses telephone interviews with children and their family members, and these researchers warn that the method "ran the risk of missing those children who were most vulnerable to being exposed either to violence in general or to specific types of violence" (Hamby et al., 2011, p. 5). Parents who do expose their children to PIPV may not be willing to discuss these events with a stranger over the telephone. For this reason, a truly representative national sample that accurately depicts these kinds of experiences may not be attainable. Similarly, clinical samples are problematic, but they may be taking the right approach in that these studies locate populations of children who tend to exhibit the outcomes of abuse and then inquire about prior abuse within those populations. This strategy might be necessary to fully understand the dynamics of abuse and its aftereffects, but it is important to recognize that most people who do experience bad parenting do not grow up committing serious crimes. Another accessible population of youth who tend to exhibit many of the outcomes of abuse is incarcerated youth, and this population is significantly larger and more accessible to researchers than most clinical samples and may not be as prone to social class biases.

Measures of Family Violence

For the past 14 years or so, it has been generally accepted that the types of abuses that children are exposed to in the household are multidimensional (Holt et al., 2008). They include personal abuses that children experience as physical, sexual, or emotional assaults and neglect as well as exposure to these forms of PIPV. Abusive experiences often coexist in the same household (Edleson, 1999). Many measurement advances were made in the 1980s and 1990s regarding the conceptualization of exposure (Cunningham & Baker, 2004; Mullender et al., 2002). Children can witness parental abuse directly, overhear the abusive situation, or simply learn about it after its occurrence by seeing its physical effects, such as bruises or broken dishes. Types of exposure to PIPV are hierarchical in this manner from most to least serious experiences.

THE OCEAN TIDES STUDY AND VIOLENCE

The methods and database construction for the Ocean Tides study were explained in the previous chapter. Briefly then, the database contains 1,585 cases of boys who entered the Ocean Tides program from 1975 to 2006. This research addresses several of the shortcomings in the existing literature on the effects of personal child abuse and exposure to PIPV and their effects on violent behavior. First, the Ocean Tides data come from multiple sources: self-reports, parent surveys, social worker reports, police reports and juvenile court records, teachers, school records, and the clinical interviews that are explained in detail in Chapter 8. It does not rely on a single source for information.

In this study, we have lifetime measures of exposure to PIPV, the juvenile's personal abusive victimization, and measures of his own violent behavior prior to and while residing in Ocean Tides. We use accepted practices from the literature by considering different types of exposure to PIPV—witnessing, overhearing, and otherwise knowing about it—and we developed measures that account for the hierarchical nature of these experiences. Three types of personal child abuse and exposure to PIPV are measured: physical, sexual, and emotional.

Exposure to PIPV Measures in the Ocean Tides Study

We use a contemporary and practical definition of parents. Parental figures come in all configurations: biological parents; stepparents who are married to a biological parent or cohabitating; part-time-live-in boyfriends and girlfriends; extended relatives who play the role of parental figures, such as aunts, uncles, grandparents, and older siblings; foster parents; and other guardians. We define a parental figure as anyone who even temporarily served in that role for the boy in his lifetime. "Stepparent" is defined as one being married to a biological parent, and "other-parent" includes anyone else except biological parents.

Children are exposed to different kinds of abuse among parental figures: physical, sexual, and emotional. Physical abuse among parental figures includes any physical violence whether or not it resulted in visible physical harm, but which is generally unwanted physical (but not sexual) contact between parents. In our study, this includes both simple (no external weapon involved) and aggravated (use of a weapon) assaults. Although it is rare even in our study for a child to be exposed to sexual violence between parents, we do find 10 cases. Sexual abuse is not also measured as a form of physical abuse. Although experiencing physical and/or sexual abuse is emotionally abusive, our measure of emotional abuse includes only incidents of it that occur separate from any physical or sexual PIPV. Emotional abuse is often expressed by a pattern of verbal threats or insults or excessively manipulative behavior by parents in this study.

For each type and manner in which the boys are exposed to PIPV, we measure frequency as (a) only being exposed to a single isolated event in his lifetime; (b) a few times; or (c) often, for each parental partnership. To create our final variables for analyses, we wanted to capture the intensity of exposure so that boys who witnessed abuse, for example, had higher scores on PIPV exposure than boys who overheard it, also taking frequency of exposure into account. First, working just with "witnessed" "physical" violence, we combined exposure by all parental figures by adding scores together so that someone who was exposed only once by each of three different combinations of parental figures, for example, would have a score of "3" on the new variable. Likewise, someone who was exposed repeatedly by the same couple and no others would have the same score. We did the same thing to create interval variables for physical PIPV exposure that was overheard and otherwise known about as separate measures. Then, to capture the hierarchy among witnessing, overhearing, or otherwise knowing about physical PIPV exposure, we combined these variables so that witnessed exposure was weighted by "3," overheard by "2," and otherwise "known about" by "1." Our final physical PIPV exposure variable includes 19 points that range from 1 (no exposure at all) to a score of 43.

We used the same procedure to create a final emotional PIPV exposure variable that includes 12 points that range from 1 (no exposure at all) to a score of 18 and a variable for sexual PIPV exposure that includes 6 points and ranges from 1 to 13. Dichotomous variables were also created (1 = no exposure and 2 = exposure) for each type of exposure to PIPV.

The boys in our sample are slightly more likely than boys in the general population to be exposed to physical PIPV (Figure 4.1). Hamby et al. (2011) report lifetime rates of exposure to physical PIPV for boys from the only representative national sample of youth in the United States as 16.9%, while 18.5% ($n = 294$) of the Ocean Tides boys were exposed to it. Comparisons between national samples and our sample for emotional abuse are more challenging because we can assume that only the most pervasive exposure to emotional PIPV would find its way into the boys' files at Ocean Tides. The Hamby et al. (2011) study found that 14.7% of boys are exposed to emotional PIPV, whereas in our sample, it is 6.7% ($n = 106$). It is reasonable to believe that these differences may be due to methodology and sampling effects because similar definitions of emotional abuse are used in both studies. Ten boys (0.6%) were exposed to sexual PIPV, and this type of PIPV is considered so remote that it is not even calculated in national samples.

It is interesting to note that in the early stages of the Ocean Tides project, the researchers were repeatedly turned down for national funding because, on each request, they were told that it was common knowledge that every young man in the legal system was probably exposed

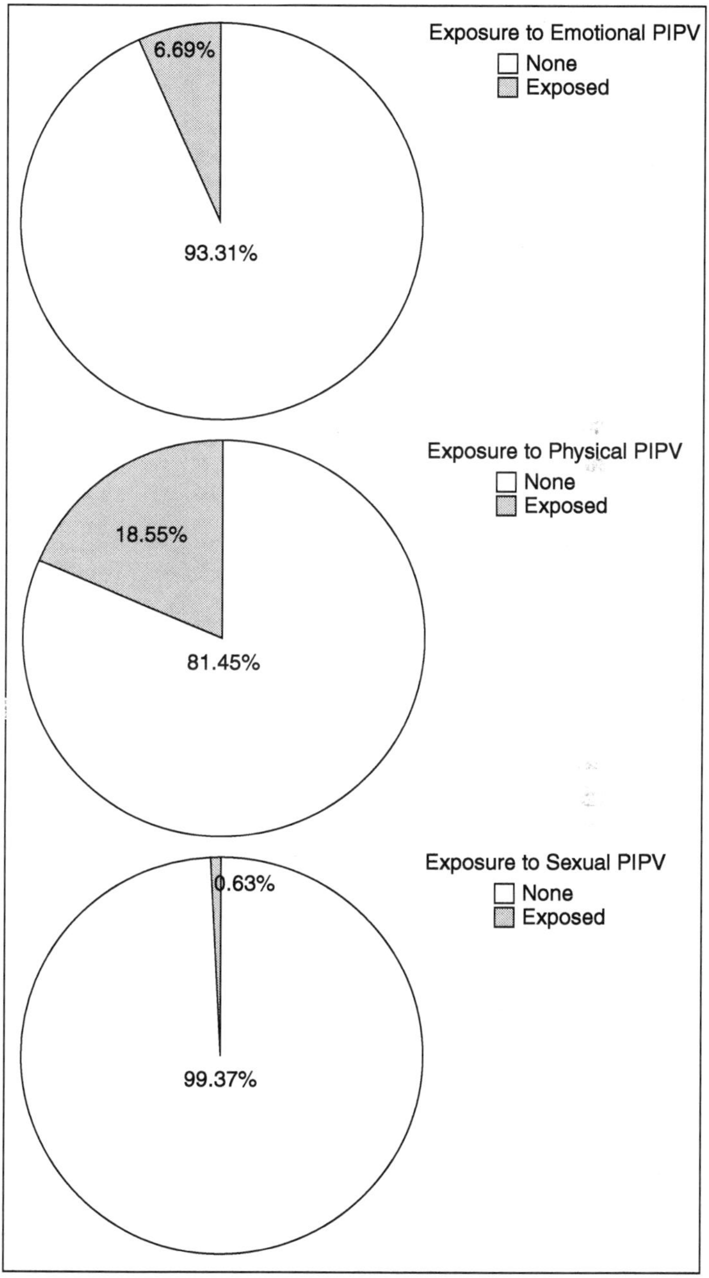

FIGURE 4.1 Lifetime exposure to parental interpersonal violence (PIPV).

to PIPV at some point in his lifetime. Despite repeated attempts, the researchers could not convince the funding agencies that they were relying on and reiterating stereotypes that had never been empirically replicated. Although exposure to PIPV is a very important problem, care should always be taken not to overexaggerate its prevalence in any particular population.

The boys in our study were most often exposed to abuse that was perpetrated by father figures against their maternal figures. Six percent of the Ocean Tides boys were exposed to emotional abuse by fathers against mothers and 4.3% were exposed to female-to-male parental emotional abuse. Twenty-one percent of the boys were exposed to physical PIPV perpetrated by fathers against mothers compared to 1.2% of mothers against fathers. Biological fathers were the perpetrators of sexual violence against mothers in all 10 cases of exposure. Ironically, the absence of a father figure is viewed as negative, but these situations question this cultural assumption, at least for many of the Ocean Tides boys.

Personal Child Abuse Measures in the Ocean Tides Study

Our measures of personal child abuse that is directly experienced by the juvenile include all perpetrators: parental figures, siblings, and other relatives and nonrelatives in the home. We measure physical, emotional, and sexual abuse. For each abusive event per child, it is measured only as one type of abuse; so, for example, sexual or physical abuse is not also recorded as emotional even though there are obvious emotional repercussions from these other forms of violence. The frequency of abuse is measured as (a) a single isolated event, (b) a few times, or (3) often.

For our final abuse variables, we summed all scores from all sources for each type of abuse to create three measures of abuse. Physical abuse has 13 scores that range from 1 (no physical abuse) to 18, with higher scores indicating more serious abuse (more sources and/or greater frequency of abuse). Sexual abuse has eight scores that range from 1 to 9, and emotional abuse has 15 scores that range from 1 to 15, with intensity patterns similar to the physical abuse variable.

Child abuse statistics are presented in Figure 4.2. Nearly 55% ($n = 869$) of the boys in this study experienced emotional abuse in their lifetimes, 23.5% ($n = 372$) of the boys were physically abused, and 6.2%

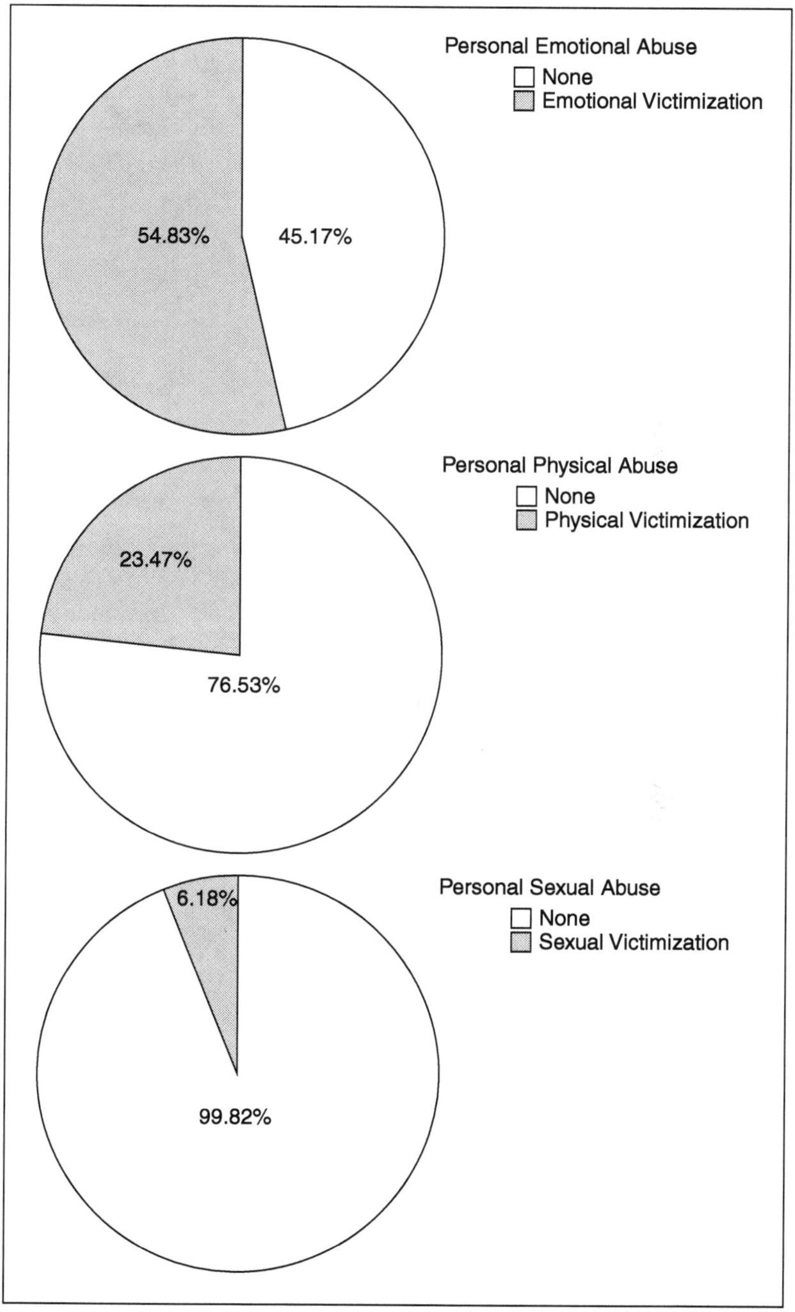

FIGURE 4.2 Lifetime measures of personal child abuse.

(n = 98) were sexually abused. The U.S. Department of Health and Human Services (2013) offers national estimates that dramatically differ from ours: 8.5% of youth were psychologically abused, 18.3% were physically abused, and 9.3% were sexually abused. These national statistics are based on abuses that are reported to officials and our data include those and abuses that are not reported. Furthermore, ours is a sample of offenders who exhibit many of the outcomes of abuse; so it stands to reason that these figures differ.

Violent Behavior Measures in the Ocean Tides Study

We create four measures of violent behavior from all sources in the database combined (see the previous chapter for an explanation of data sources). Two are continuous with low scores that indicate no problem or a minor problem and higher scores mean more severe problems. Two other variables are dichotomous: (a) no violence and (b) violent behavior. One continuous and one dichotomous variable represent violent behavior prior to entering the Ocean Tides program and the other two represent violent behavior during the boy's stay in the facility. The continuous measures of violence are presented as (a) no indication of a problem at all, (b) a slight problem (one or two incidents), (c) a moderate problem, and (d) a severe problem.

Prior to Ocean Tides, about 58% of the boys behaved violently compared to approximately 21% while they were residing in the facility (Figure 4.3). Recall that the boys are not on lockdown while at Ocean Tides, and they are allowed to go home for weekends, extended passes on holidays, and school vacations. Their behavior on weekend leave is assessed by parent interviews, self-reports, and reports from social workers. Even so, severe violence decreases 43.45%: from 46.86% of the boys before they went to Ocean Tides to 3.41% while the boys are in the care of the program.

EXPOSURE TO PIPV, PERSONAL CHILD ABUSE, AND VIOLENCE

Roughly one fifth of the boys who had behaved violently prior to entering Ocean Tides experienced some form of personal child abuse and were exposed to PIPV. Table 4.1 contains a lot of valuable and interesting

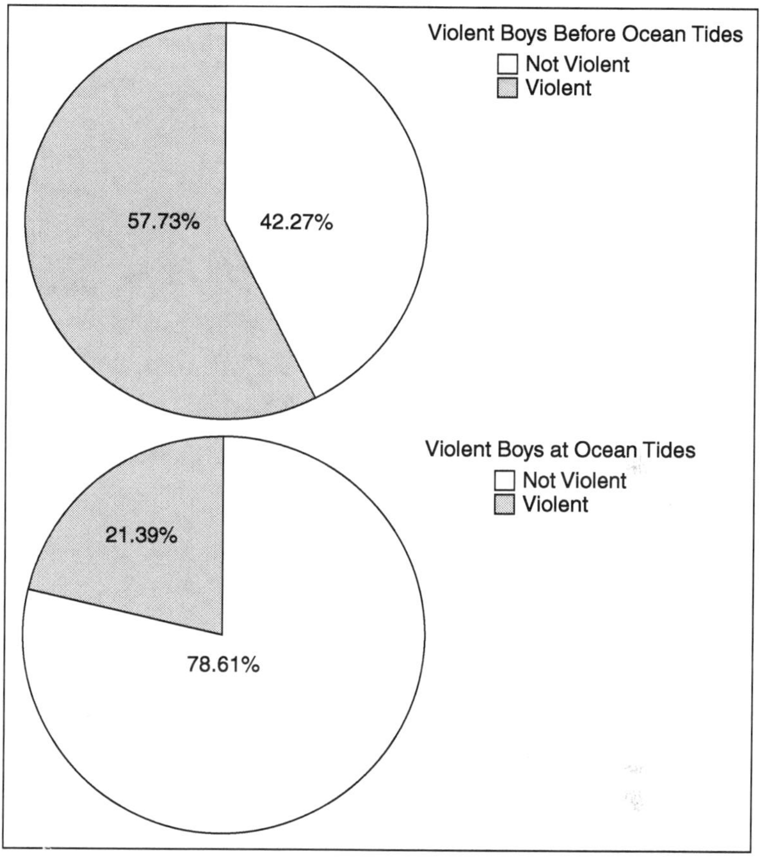

FIGURE 4.3 Violent behavior before Ocean Tides, and while residing in Ocean Tides.

information about change in patterns of violence. Chi-square analyses identified statistically significant differences between violent and nonviolent boys for each type of abuse and exposure to PIPV prior to entering Ocean Tides. However, there were no significant differences in violent behavior while residing in Ocean Tides between boys who had previously been exposed to any type of PIPV and those who had not. This means that although exposure does increase the likelihood of violence before entering the program, the effects lose their impact on violence while residing in the facility. These are lifetime measures of exposure, too, which means that we are not simply removing the boys from current violent situations. These results imply that their

TABLE 4.1
Victimized Boys Who Were Also Violent

	PERSONAL ABUSE			EXPOSURE TO PIPV		
VICTIMIZATION	Before OT (%)	At OT (%)	Decrease in Violence (%)	Before OT	At OT	Decrease in Violence (%)
Emotional	61.4 (10.916**)	24.2 (8.828*)	61	74.5 (13.138***)	20.8 (.028)	72
Physical	67.2 (17.885***)	28.5 (14.601***)	58	68.4 (16.741***)	23.8 (1.259)	65
Sexual	78.6 (18.596***)	38.8 (18.783***)	51	90 (4.295*)	30 (.444)	67

Note: Percentages in the before and at OT columns are the percentage of boys who experienced abuse or exposure in their lifetimes and behaved violently either before entering the OT program or while they were in residence. Numbers in parentheses are chi-square results and *p* values. All analyses include all cases ($n = 1{,}585$).

OT, Ocean Tides; PIPV, parental interpersonal violence.

*$p < .05$. **$p < .01$. ***$p < .000$.

experiences in the Ocean Tides program lessen the long-term effects of exposure to PIPV.

Table 4.1 also contains data that represent the percentage of boys who experienced abuse or exposure in their lifetimes and behaved violently either before or after entering the Ocean Tides program. For example, 61.4% of boys who experienced personal emotional abuse were violent prior to entering Ocean Tides, whereas only 24.2% of them remained violent while residing in the program. We see a drastic decrease in violence at Ocean Tides for boys who experienced every type of personal abuse and every type of exposure to PIPV. Although boys who were victims of personal abuse were still more likely than non victims to be violent at Ocean Tides, fewer of these boys continued to act violently once they got into the program.

We further conducted two sets of multivariate analyses: one in which we looked at the effects of the presence of violence in the boys' lives on the likelihood that the boys will act violently. Second, we looked at the effects of the intensity of violence in the boys' lives on the intensity of their own violent behavior before and after entering Ocean Tides. We included demographic characteristics and control for the effects of prior violent behavior on violent behavior while at Ocean Tides.

What Increases the Likelihood of Violent Behavior?

Using only the dichotomous variables—no abuse versus abuse—we test if the presence of violence in the boys' lives increases the likelihood that the boys will act violently. Bivariate coefficients are shown in Table 4.2 and indicate that all three forms of violent abuse experienced by the boys and all three forms of exposure to PIPV independently significantly increase the likelihood that a boy behaved violently prior to entering the Ocean Tides program. However, while residing in the Ocean Tides program, the effects of exposure to PIPV on violence wane.

Interestingly, we find that sexual abuse and each of the three forms of exposure to PIPV are not correlated; so boys who experience this type of abuse are not also more likely to be exposed to PIPV. However, all of the other forms of abuse and exposure to PIPV are significantly correlated, as we would expect. This means that boys who are exposed to physical or emotional PIPV are also more likely to be personally physically or emotionally abused. Recall that our measures of emotional abuse are independent of any other type of abuse the boys experience; so the emotional abuse a boy receives from others is not measured as a direct component or result of the physical or sexual abuse he receives.

Race and violence are significantly correlated, such that non-White boys are more likely to act violently in our study than White boys (Pearson's r = .064* [asterisks defined in footnote to Table 4.3]), but violence is not related to SES (Pearson's r = –.009). White boys are significantly higher in SES than are non-White youth in this study (Pearson's r = –.178**). SES also varies for some of the victimization that the boys experience. Those with higher SES are more likely to experience emotional abuse (Pearson's r = –.130**) and are at greater risk of being exposed to sexual PIPV (Pearson's r = –.054*). Race is also correlated with some of the violence experienced by the boys. White youth are at greater risk of exposure to physical PIPV (Pearson's r = –.081**) and emotional PIPV (Pearson's r = –.082**). They are also more likely to be physically (Pearson's r = –.095**) and sexually (Pearson's r = –.069*) abused.

Logistic regression models were constructed guided by the bivariate results and are presented in Table 4.3. One model tests the effects of violent exposure to PIPV and abuse on the boys' violent behavior prior to entering the Ocean Tides facility, and the second model tests these effects on youth violence while the boys were part of the program.

TABLE 4.2
Pearson's Correlation Coefficients for Dichotomous Variables

	1	2	3	4	5	6	7	8	9
1. Physical abuse									
2. Emotional abuse	.216**								
3. Sexual abuse	.130**	.091**							
4. Physical PIPV	.337**	.140**	.046						
5. Emotional PIPV	.197**	.147**	.036	.360**					
6. Sexual PIPV	.106**	.072**	.013	.146**	.170**				
7. Violence	.106**	.083**	.108**	.103**	.091**	.052*			
8. Violence at OT	.096**	.075**	.109**	.028	–.004	.017	.191**		
9. Race	–.095**	–.043	–.069*	–.081**	–.082**	–.036	.064*	.010	
10. SES	–.004	–.130**	.018	–.028	.017	–.054*	–.009	–.016	–.178**

OT, Ocean Tides; PIPV, parental interpersonal violence; SES, socioeconomic status.

*$p \leq .05$ and **$p \leq .01$; $n = 1{,}585$.

TABLE 4.3
Logistic Regression Analyses of Variables Predicting Violent Behavior Before (n = 1,323) and While Residing in OT (n = 1,585)

PREDICTOR	VIOLENT BEHAVIOR PRIOR TO OT			VIOLENT BEHAVIOR WHILE RESIDING AT OT		
	B	SE B	e^B	B	SE B	e^B
Emotional abuse	.12	.11	1.13	.21	.13	1.23
Physical abuse	.37**	.15	1.45	.31*	.14	1.37
Sexual abuse	.97***	.28	2.63	.64**	.22	1.89
Emotional PIPV	.47	.26	1.60			
Physical PIPV	.33*	.17	1.40			
Sexual PIPV	1.19	1.08	3.31			
Race	.38***	.11	1.46			
Violence before OT				.95***	.14	2.58
Constant	−3.93			−4.29		
χ^2		56.66			80.63	
df		7			4	

Race: 1 = White; 2 = non-White. e^B= exponentiated B.
OT, Ocean Tides; PIPV, parental interpersonal violence; SE, standard error.
*$p \leq .05$. **$p \leq .01$. ***$p \leq .001$.

Both models are statistically significant. The first model includes all three forms of exposure to PIPV, personal child abuses, and race. As race is included in the first model, that analysis contains 1,323 cases, whereas the second model includes all cases (n = 1,585). SES was not correlated with either measure of the boys' violent behaviors and so it is not included in either model. The second model includes no measures of exposure to PIPV or race because these variables were not significantly correlated with violence while residing in Ocean Tides; but this second model does take into account the effects of the boy's prior violent behavior on current violence. The best predictor of future violence is past violence; so it is common practice in research to include this measure in multivariate analyses.

Partial coefficients in the first model indicate that while controlling for the effects of the other variables in the model, violent behavior prior to Ocean Tides increases with the experience of physical abuse (p = .013), sexual abuse (p = .001), and exposure to physical PIPV (p = .048).

The effects of sexual abuse have the strongest influence on violent behavior—slightly stronger than the effects of race (p = .001). Non-White youth remain more likely to act violently than Whites even while controlling for the effects of the other variables in the model.

In the second model, controlling for the effects of the other variables, violent behavior while in the Ocean Tides program continues to be significantly influenced by prior physical abuse (p = .027) and sexual abuse (p = .004). The strongest correlation, however, is the effect of the boy's prior violent behavior on his behavior at Ocean Tides (p = .000). This effect is independent of the effects of exposure to PIPV and the other abuses he has endured in his lifetime. This result implies that violence may become a force of habit over time that takes on a life of its own, separate from its original causes.

What Increases the Intensity of Violent Behavior?

Our second set of analyses examines how the intensity of exposure to violence affects the intensity of violent behavior. By intensity, we mean how frequently violent behavior occurs combined with how serious the events are in terms of the harm they inflict. Cuevas et al. (2013) conclude that "factoring in repeated victimizations and other measures of victimization severity does not produce substantively different results in identifying highly victimized youth" (Finkelhor, Ormrod, & Turner, 2007; Finkelhor, Turner, Ormond, & Hamby, 2005). Nonetheless, some studies do find that it makes a difference, and our sample is unique enough to merit its inclusion.

Table 4.4 contains Pearson's correlation coefficients for bivariate relationships among the continuous variables. Prior to entering the Ocean Tides program, greater intensity of each of the three forms of exposure to PIPV and each of the three forms of personal abuse increases the intensity of violent behavior. The intensity of violence while residing in Ocean Tides is increased by all but exposure to emotional PIPV.

Similar to results for the likelihood of violence, we find that the intensity of sexual abuse experiences and at least two of the three forms of exposure to PIPV are not correlated: physical and sexual exposure to PIPV. However, unlike the previous analysis, it is significantly correlated with exposure to emotional PIPV (Pearson's r = .050*). All of the other forms of abuse and exposure are correlated with each of the

TABLE 4.4
Pearson's Correlation Coefficients for Continuous Variables

CONTINUOUS VARIABLE	1	2	3	4	5	6	7	8	9
1. Physical abuse									
2. Emotional abuse	.361**								
3. Sexual abuse	.211**	.153**							
4. Physical PIPV	.329**	.185**	.041						
5. Emotional PIPV	.187**	.192**	.050*	.426**					
6. Sexual PIPV	.153**	.061*	–.002	.297**	.175**				
7. Violence	.104**	.071**	.108**	.125**	.077**	.050*			
8. Violence at OT	.153**	.110**	.111**	.083**	.016	.064*	.161**		
9. Race	–.077**	–.090**	–.062*	–.051	–.071**	.010	.093**	.025	
10. SES	–.029	–.055*	.038	–.043	.019	–.058*	–.015	–.038	–.178**

OT, Ocean Tides; PIPV, parental interpersonal violence; SES, socioeconomic status.

$*p \leq .05$. $**p \leq .01$. $n = 1,585$.

TABLE 4.5
Simple Analyses of Variables Predicting Violent Behavior Before (n = 1,322) and While (n = 1,584) Residing in OT

PREDICTOR	VIOLENT BEHAVIOR PRIOR TO OT			VIOLENT BEHAVIOR WHILE RESIDING IN OT		
	B	SE B	β	B	SE B	β
Emotional abuse	.01	.02	.02	.01	.01	.04
Physical abuse	.04	.02	.05	.05	.01	.10***
Sexual abuse	.22	.06	.09***	.09	.03	.06**
Emotional PIPV	.01	.01	.02			
Physical PIPV	.02	.01	.09**	.00	.00	.00
Sexual PIPV	.03	.08	.01	.07	.04	.04
Race	.32	.07	.11***			
Violence before OT				.07	.01	.13***
R^2		.04			.05	
F		8.39***			14.87***	

OT, Ocean Tides; PIPV, parental interpersonal violence; SE, standard error.
Race: 1 = White, 2 = non-White.
$^{**}p \leq .01$. $^{***}p \leq .001$.

others; so overall, boys who experience one form of abuse or exposure are also more likely to experience others. These results confirm prior research on polyvictimization.

Non-White boys exhibit more intense violence than White boys prior to entering Ocean Tides (Pearson's r = .093**), but that relationship disappears at Ocean Tides. SES does not affect the intensity of violence either before or at Ocean Tides. White boys endure more intense physical abuse (Pearson's r = −.077**), emotional abuse (Pearson's r = −.090**), sexual abuse (Pearson's r = −.062*), and are exposed to more intense parental emotional PIPV (Pearson's r = −.071**) than non-White boys. Boys from lower SES experience more intense emotional abuse (Pearson's r = −.055*) and are exposed to more sexual PIPV (Pearson's r = −.058*).

Two models are tested using ordinary least squares (OLS) linear regression (Table 4.5). Both models are statistically significant. As the first model excludes those for whom we have no measure of race, it contains 1,322 cases and the second model includes the whole sample (n = 1,584). The first model includes all of the violence variables prior to Ocean Tides and race. Controlling for the effects of the other variables in the model, the intensity of violent behavior prior to Ocean Tides is increased by more intense victimization by sexual abuse (p = .001), exposure to physical PIPV (p = .004), and race, such that non-Whites engage in more intense violence prior to entering the program.

In the second model, we examine what increases the intensity of violent behavior while residing in the Ocean Tides facility. This model excludes variables that were not significantly correlated with the violence in the bivariate analyses: emotional abuse, race, and SES. It includes all other variables, including a measure of the intensity of violence prior to entering Ocean Tides. Controlling for other effects in the model, increased intensity of prior physical abuse (p = .000), prior sexual abuse (p = .008), and the intensity of prior violence behavior (p = .000) significantly increases the intensity of violence after the boys enter the Ocean Tides program.

CONCLUSIONS

So much less is understood about exposure to PIPV than what we already know about the dangerous effects of other forms of child abuse. The current study opens inroads toward greater understanding about this complex experience that adds unnecessary stress to children's lives. Until now, no research has tested the long-term effects of exposure to PIPV and how those effects may be ameliorated by removing the child from the abusive home. Most studies confound violent behavior with more general aggression; so little is known about what causes violence. The Ocean Tides study addresses several shortcomings in the existing body of research on exposure to PIPV by using a large sample with information from multiple sources in these boys' lives. The current study also utilizes accepted practices for defining and measuring exposure to PIPV.

Before being sent to the Ocean Tides program, well over half of the boys behaved violently. In the program, only 21% of them were violent. We find that boys who were exposed to PIPV before entering the program were much more likely to act violently and their violence was much more intense than that of those who were not exposed; however, once they entered the program, the effects of those noxious experiences on violence diminished. Hence, the long-term effects of exposure may be weakened by the right kinds of intervention that involve the removal of the boy from his current environment. As exposure to PIPV and direct child abuse often occur together, where one is present, the child should be removed from the home.

We find that prior to entering Ocean Tides, boys who were physically or sexually abused or boys who were exposed to physical PIPV were most likely to act violently. Prior to Ocean Tides, non-White youth were more likely to act violently and they engaged in more intense forms of violence, but racial differences disappear at Ocean Tides. This finding indicates that the often-cited correlation between race and violence may indeed be due to factors other than race itself because the boys' biological makeup does not change when they enter the Ocean Tides program. The presence of past violent behavior and its intensity are the strongest predictors of violent behavior at Ocean Tides, and although the effects of prior physical and sexual abuse are diminished in the program, they remain important predictors. The effects of exposure to PIPV on violent behavior at Ocean Tides disappear.

Removing a child from an abusive environment is one important piece of the puzzle, but where do they go, especially if they are already behaving badly? Geffner, Igelman, and Zellner (2003, p. 5) argue that one of the most effective intervention strategies for ameliorating the ill effects of exposure to PIPV is when support people "act as surrogate parents." Bad parenting is only one source of potential strain in a young man's life. Another source is what is missing from his life: the absence of positive parenting. The Ocean Tides program aims to provide that role: to identify the missing pieces of their lives and lay inroads toward making them whole.

REFERENCES

Agnew, R. (2005). *Why do criminals offend? A general theory of crime and delinquency.* Los Angeles, CA: Roxbury.

Appel, A. E., & Holden, G. W. (1998). The co-occurrence of spouse and physical child abuse: A review and appraisal. *Journal of Family Psychology, 12*(4), 578–599.

Baldry, A. C. (2003). Bullying in schools and exposure to domestic violence. *Child Abuse and Neglect, 27*, 713–732.

Cuevas, C. A., Finkelhor, D., Shattuck, A., Turner, H., & Hamby, S. (2013). Children's exposure to violence and the intersection between delinquency and victimization. *Juvenile Justice Bulletin: OJJDP National Survey of Children's*

Exposure to Violence. Washington, DC: U.S. Department of Justice, Office of Justice Programs.

Cunningham, A., & Baker, L. (2004). *What about me! Seeking to understand a child's view of violence in the family.* London, Ontario: Centre for Children and Families in the Justice System.

Edleson, J. L. (1999). Children's witnessing of adult domestic violence. *Journal of Interpersonal Violence, 14*(8), 839–870.

Ehrensaft, M. K., Cohen, P., Brown, J., Smailes, E., Chen, H., & Johnson, J. G. (2003). Intergenerational transmission of partner violence: A 20-year prospective study. *Journal of Consulting and Clinical Psychology, 71*(4), 741–753.

Finkelhor, D., Ormrod, R., & Turner, H. (2007). Polyvictimization and trauma in a national longitudinal cohort. *Development and Psychopathology, 19*, 149–166.

Finkelhor, D., Turner, H., Ormrod, R., & Hamby, S. L. (2005). The victimization of children and youth: A comprehensive, national survey. *Child Maltreatment, 10*(1), 5–25.

Geffner, R. A., Igelman, R. S., & Zellner, J. (2003). Introduction: Children exposed to interparental violence: A need for additional research and validated treatment programs. In R. A. Geffner, R. S. Igelman, & J. Zellner (Eds.), *The effects of intimate partner violence on children* (pp. 1–10). New York, NY: The Haworth Maltreatment and Trauma Press.

Hamby, S., Finkelhor, D., Turner, H., & Ormrod, R. (2011). Children's exposure to intimate partner violence and other family violence. *Juvenile Justice Bulletin: OJJDP National Survey of Children's Exposure to Violence.* Washington, DC: U.S. Department of Justice, Office of Justice Programs.

Holden, G. W. (2003). Children exposed to domestic violence and child abuse: Terminology and taxonomy. *Clinical Child and Family Psychological Review, 6*(3), 151–160.

Holt, S., Buckley, H., & Whelan, S. (2008). The impact of exposure to domestic violence on children and young people: A review of the literature. *Child Abuse and Neglect, 32*, 797–810.

Jaffe, P. G., Wolfe, D. A., Wilson, S. K., & Zak, L. (1986). Similarities in behavioral and social maladjustment among child victims and witnesses to family violence. *American Journal of Orthopsychiatry, 56*(1), 142–146.

Jouriles, E. N., McDonald, R., Norwood, W. D., Ware, S. H., Spiller, L. C., & Swank, P. R. (1998). Knives, guns, and interparent violence: Relations with child behavior problems. *Journal of Family Psychology, 12*(2), 178–194.

Kerig, P. K. (1998). Gender and appraisals as mediators of adjustment in children exposed to interparental violence. *Developmental Psychology, 29*(6), 931–939.

Lewis, C. E., Siegel, J. M., & Lewis, M. A. (1984). Feeling bad: Exploring sources of distress among pre-adolescent children. *American Journal of Public Health, 74*, 117–122.

McDonald, R., Jouriles, E. N., Norwood, W., Ware, H. S., & Ezell, E. (2000). Husbands' marital violence and the adjustment problems of clinic-referred children. *Behavior Therapy, 31*, 649–665.

Mullender, A., Hague, G., Iman, U., Kelly, L., Malos, E., & Regan, L. (2002). *Children's perspectives on domestic violence*. London, England: Sage Publications.

Murrell, A. R., Merwin, R. M., Christoff, K. A., & Henning, K. R. (2005). When parents model violence: The relationship between witnessing weapon use as a child and later use as an adult. *Behavior and Social Issues, 14*, 128–133.

O'Keefe, M. (1994). Adjustment of children from maritally violent homes. *Families in Society: The Journal of Contemporary Human Services, 75*(7), 403–415.

Onyskiw, J. E. (2003). Domestic violence and children's adjustment: A review of research. *Journal of Emotional Abuse, 3*(1/2), 11–15.

Osofsky, J. D. (1999). The impact of violence on children. *The Future of Children, 9*(3), 33–49.

Steinberg, L. (2000). Youth violence: Do parents and families make a difference? *National Institute of Justice Journal, 2*, 30–38.

Stith, S. M., Rosen, K. H., Middleton, K. A., Busch, A. L., Lundeberg, K., & Carlton, R. P. (2000). The intergenerational transmission of spouse abuse: A meta-analysis. *Journal of Marriage and Family, 62*(3), 640–654.

U.S. Department of Health and Human Services, Administration for Children and Families, Children's Bureau. (2013). *Child maltreatment, 2012*. Retrieved from http://www.acf.hhs.gov/sites/default/files/cb/cm2012.pdf

Wekerle, C., & Wolfe, D. A. (1999). Dating violence in mid-adolescence: Theory, significance, and emerging prevention initiatives. *Clinical Psychological Review, 19*(4), 435–456.

CHAPTER 5

Charting a Course: The Program at Ocean Tides

The Ocean Tides program is organized into five main components: education, group living (residential life), social services, the extension houses, and aftercare. For many years, there was a community-based early intervention diversionary program that targeted youngsters at high risk for juvenile offenses. This program was discontinued when Tides Family Services, a nonprofit, community-based multiservice program developed by a former president of Ocean Tides, replaced it. The education component consists of a fully accredited high school with a staff of experienced teachers. The school also has a Providence Campus for residents at the extension houses, former residents in aftercare, youngsters who have completed the program but cannot return to public school, and tuition-based youngsters referred by their municipal school districts. The group-living segment involves supervision of the young men when they are not in school, including recreational activities and residential life. Social services consists of graduate-trained clinical social workers who provide individual and family counseling, liaison with the youngsters' families and community resources, and a variety of support services. They also maintain contact with youngsters during the 3 months of aftercare that follows completion of the program. In the aftercare component, youngsters who have successfully completed the program are followed by a social worker in order to facilitate their successful reintegration to the community.

PROGRAM ADMINISTRATION

Each program component has its own director who reports to the president. The president serves as the overall director of treatment. Together, these administrators comprise the administrative team and are responsible for the administration of the program. The administrative team consists of the president, director of administration, director of education (principal of the school), assistant principal in charge of the Providence Campus, director of special education, director of social services, director of residential life (group living), and directors of the extension houses and honor dorm. The administrative team meets regularly to make practical decisions regarding disciplinary procedures and other decisions about the day-to-day running of the program. The president is responsible for overall administration of the program, including budget management and development, external funding, and liaison with state and federal agencies.

The director of administration/quality improvement officer (QIO) reports directly to the president/executive director and is responsible for the administrative operation and regulatory compliance of the Ocean Tides program. The position consists of three specific roles: QIO, corporate compliance officer (CCO), and assistant to the president. The specific responsibilities of the QIO are to coordinate the organization's reaccreditation and compliance with standards for several accrediting agencies, including Commission on Accreditation of Rehabilitation Facilities (CARF); New England Association of Schools and Colleges (NEASC); and the Prison Rape Elimination Act (PREA). Additional responsibilities include developing and managing the organization's strategic plan, risk management plan, accessibility plan, technology plan, and quality improvement plan/report. The responsibilities of the CCO are to direct and manage the organization's compliance with the Rhode Island Department of Children, Youth and Families (DCYF) Residential Child Care Regulations; Medicaid reimbursement regulations, including federal and state laws that pertain to organizations that receive federal and state funds; Health Insurance Portability and Accountability Act (HIPAA); and all other applicable regulations. Implementing these responsibilities involves a number of more specific duties within the organization.

STAFF DEVELOPMENT AND EVALUATION

A key to the success of the Ocean Tides program is to identify and hire good people and help them get better at their jobs by providing ongoing opportunities for in-service training, close supervision, and the close monitoring of job performance. The administration recognizes the value and importance of providing professional training and personal support for staff on a regular basis. Staff development is provided in several ways: by the regular dissemination of articles and information related to the rehabilitation of troubled youngsters; development of departmental libraries that include relevant books and periodical literature; opportunities for staff to visit other programs and agencies to observe alternative approaches; the provision of both department-specific and program-wide in-service education and workshops on selected topics by outside consultants and other experts; the opportunity to meet with the consulting psychologist on an individual basis to discuss how to deal with difficult situations, work-related stress, and problems with residents; and by weekly departmental staff meetings that may be attended by an outside consultant. These weekly departmental staff meetings are particularly important for staff development and support. They are devoted to discussions of current problems with an individual youngster or other issues, sharing of personal frustrations and stress related to work, discussion of interpersonal conflicts and differences of opinion among staff, and mediation of conflicts. Working with delinquents is an emotionally demanding and highly stressful occupation. Consequently, staff members are vulnerable to both "burn out" and conflict with each other. Creating an environment in which the emotional welfare of the staff is considered a high priority helps maintain good morale and effective job performance. One of the most important functions of an outside consultant is to serve as a facilitator for staff to express and share their frustrations, anger, disappointments, and other troublesome emotions in an open, candid, and self-disclosing manner at staff meetings.

Department heads provide evaluation of regular staff on an informal but regular basis through feedback and discussion. The evaluation of department heads is more structured and the outside consultant conducts a formal written evaluation of every department head on a yearly basis. This evaluation consists of two parts: the staff members anonymously complete a 20-item 5-rating Likert-type scale and the opportunity to add individual written comments; and meet as a group with the outside consultant to discuss the administrator's performance during the past year. The consultant takes detailed notes of the staff members' comments, including notable quotes. After collecting the data, the consultant summarizes the ratings, written comments (including verbatim), and oral comments. The consultant then prepares a written report based on the staff's written and oral input and submits it to the president. All administrators have the opportunity to read, discuss, and react to their annual evaluations. Appendix B contains a copy of the evaluation form and Appendix C contains sample reports.

TREATMENT TEAMS

Each resident is assigned to a treatment team consisting of one staff member each from the education, group living, and social services components. The treatment team is responsible for developing and implementing an individualized treatment plan for each boy. The primary purpose of the treatment team is to ensure that the following treatment objectives are met:

1. That there is regular and effective interdepartmental communication about a youngster's progress to ensure that he does not "slip through the cracks"
2. That each resident has specific goals and that progress toward meeting these goals is closely supervised
3. That the overall treatment plan for a boy is monitored consistently and in a practical way in each department
4. To give the resident a sense of confidence by assigning specific staff members to him whom he knows will have a special interest in him and will be particularly familiar with his situation.

Each team meets weekly with the youngster to review his progress. At the meeting, the boy is asked to review his goals and give his opinion about his progress or lack of it. The team gives feedback to the youngster about its perceptions of his progress and works out concrete steps with the boy as to how he can continue to do well or improve his behavior. The purpose of the team meeting is to review the boy's behavior, both positive and negative, and hold him accountable in order to increase his sense of personal responsibility. This is not the time or place to determine specific disciplinary actions. Individual staff members recommend specific disciplinary actions at the time that a behavioral infraction occurs. The administrative team meets on a weekly basis to review sanctions to determine if a resident has lost part or all of a weekend pass. The major purpose of the team meeting is to demonstrate the staff's concern for the resident and to encourage him to "buy into" the treatment goals as much as possible.

The staff closely monitors a resident's progress in the program. The resident's social worker has the responsibility of keeping written records of this progress as six types of reports. Brief descriptions of the types of reports and their time line follow.

1. *One-month observation*: This is essentially only a paragraph in length and includes specific behavioral observations concerning the initial adjustment of the resident and his family to the program. This report is due 30 days after the boy's date of arrival (DOA).
2. *Formal review*: There are two kinds of formal reviews. The first, called an initial treatment plan (ITP), is due 45 working days after a boy's DOA. The second, called a formal review, is due 6 months after the ITP and every 6 months thereafter. The *Social Services Department Handbook* (Ocean Tides, 1988) contains guidelines for the content and writing of these two reports.
3. *Monthly aftercare report*: All residents who complete the residential portion of the program participate in a 3-month aftercare program that is monitored by his assigned social services counselor. This report includes a summary of the resident's progress for the previous month during the aftercare phase and a list of specific goals that are being pursued.
4. *End of service report*: This report is due at the end of aftercare phase of the program. It follows the guidelines for a formal review and describes a resident's progress during aftercare. The report also provides an acceptable rationale for ending treatment.

5. *Monthly treatment notes*: These are notes that the social services counselors write once a month on each of their cases. These notes go in the resident's file and are for use only by the Ocean Tides administrators and their liaisons from the state. They are confidential and should be treated as such.
6. *Case conferences*: During the early years of the program, case conferences were held on a weekly basis. Residents, except for those on orientation, were sent home at 1 p.m. on Fridays for the weekend. This allowed staff from all departments to meet together on Friday afternoons as a full staff to discuss the residents and other program issues. The clinical psychology consultant facilitated these meetings. The purpose was to provide staff members with a more global and in-depth picture of a particular resident and to develop more effective treatment planning and implementation. Each department presented information from its perspective about the young man's history and family background, educational history and current functioning, and current adjustment to the program, including coping and relationship patterns. The staff would discuss any problems the resident might be experiencing, types of treatment strategies that had been tried with the young man, and alternative or new ways of dealing with the resident. The social services counselor whose case was being staffed at the Friday afternoon individual treatment meetings (ITMs) had the responsibility for taking notes on all the information, ideas, and treatment strategies generated at the case conference. The counselor summarized this information and presented it to the department director as soon as possible after the case conference is held, ideally within 1 month after the conference.

    These meetings allowed staff to discuss differences of opinion and also to share their own personal feelings and frustrations about their work in general and their interactions with the residents and with each other. The case conferences also provided a forum for team building, interdepartmental communication, and creating staff support. Unfortunately, the weekly meetings had to be reduced in frequency when school accreditation requirements prevented ending school early on Fridays.

CONFIDENTIALITY

Ocean Tides is a state-licensed, child care agency, and the information regarding the residents and their families is held in strictest confidence. All the young men in the program have been processed in the juvenile justice system. If, during the course of their participation in the program, the residents choose to disclose information about themselves, activities they have been involved in, incidents with the law, and/or their relationship with family members, this information must be treated confidentially. However, there is an obligation to share all pertinent information with appropriate administrators and other staff, such as department directors and social services workers. Any information that could result in physical or emotional harm to the resident or other persons is considered to be pertinent.

PROGRAM OVERSIGHT

Children's Rights to Report Suspected Abuse or Neglect

All youngsters in placement are informed of their rights to report to the proper authorities instances in which they feel there had been abusive or neglectful behavior by staff members or at home. A statement to that effect and a copy of the Children's Bill of Rights of the Rhode Island DCYF is included in the residents' handbook and is posted on a bulletin board. A resident is never denied the right to call his parents, a lawyer, or the DCYF emergency number to report alleged incidents.

Reporting of Actual or Alleged Child Abuse or Neglect

Social services counselors are in direct contact with the residents and their families. At times, there may be suspicion or evidence of child abuse or neglect. When this is the case, the following procedures are used to report actual or suspected incidents of neglect and/or abuse in accordance with the Rhode Island law. The counselor makes a verbal report followed by a written report of the situation to the director of social services. The written report includes the following information: (a) name(s) of the family members involved; (b) counselor's statement regarding whether the abuse or neglect is actual or suspected; (c) a detailed description of the type of abuse or neglect (e.g., physical, sexual, deprivation of needed care, lack of adequate supervision); (d) documentation of all observations and supporting evidence related to the alleged neglect or abuse; and (e) a description of any follow-up activities, including contacts with individuals or other agencies. When the director of social services receives a report of alleged abuse, he or she communicates this information to the treatment team. The staff member has a right to report incidents of child abuse or neglect directly to the Rhode Island DCYF.

Children's Bill of Rights

As a program under the jurisdiction of and funded by the DCYF (hereafter referred to as "the department"), Ocean Tides adheres to Rhode Island's Children's Bill of Rights. This law specifies a number of procedures designed to ensure the safety and well-being of children in treatment programs and to protect their civil rights. The bill specifies the following:

1. No child placed or treated under the supervision of the department in any public or private facility shall be deprived of any personal property or civil rights, except in accordance with due process.
2. Each child placed or treated under the supervision of the department in any public or private facility shall receive humane and dignified treatment at all times, with full respect for his personal dignity and right to privacy consistent with the treatment plan.
3. Each child placed in a secure facility under the supervision of the department shall be permitted to communicate with any individual, group, or agency, consistent with his treatment objectives; shall be provided writing materials and postage; and shall be permitted to make or receive phone calls to or from his attorneys, guardians ad litem, special advocates, or child advocate at a reasonable time.

4. The department shall adopt rules and regulations pursuant to the Administrative Procedures Act regarding children placed in secure facilities to specify the following:
   (a) When a child may be placed in restraint or seclusion or when force may be used on a child
   (b) When the head of a facility may limit the use of or receipt of mail by any child and a procedure for return of unopened mail
   (c) When the head of a facility may restrict the use of a telephone by any child.
5. A copy of any order placing a child in a secure facility under the supervision of the department in restraint or seclusion shall be made a part of the child's permanent clinical record. In addition, any special restriction on the use or receipt of mail or telephone calls shall be noted in writing, signed by the head of the facility or his designee, and made a part of the child's permanent clinical record.
6. Each child placed or treated in a secure facility under the supervision of the department shall be permitted to receive visitors subject to reasonable restriction consistent with the child's treatment plan. The head of each facility shall establish visiting hours and inform all children, their families, and other visitors of these hours. Any special restrictions shall be noted in writing, signed by the head of the facility or his designee and made a part of the child's permanent record.
7. Each child may receive his clergyman, attorney, guardian ad litem, special advocate, or child advocate at any reasonable time.
8. No person shall be denied employment, housing, civil service rank, any license or permit, including a professional license, or any other civil or legal right, solely because of a present or past placement with the department except as otherwise provided by the statute.
9. Each child under the supervision of the department shall have the right to counsel, and the right to receive visits from physicians and mental health professionals.
10. Each child shall have a right to a hearing pursuant to rules and regulations promulgated by the department if he or she is involuntarily transferred by the department to any facility outside of the state of Rhode Island in accordance with the procedure set forth in 42–72-14 of this chapter.

11. The Children's Bill of Rights shall be posted in a conspicuous place within any secure facility for the residential housing of children.
12. Every deliverer of services with whom the department enters into a purchased services agreement shall agree in writing to observe and post in a conspicuous place, the aforementioned Children's Bill of Rights.
13. Any child aggrieved by a violation of the Children's Bill of Rights may petition the Family Court for appropriate equitable relief. The Family Court shall have exclusive original jurisdiction not withstanding any remedy contained in Chapter 35 of this title.

PROGRAM STAFFING

Permanent full-time staff members provide services. In addition, there are volunteer tutors who help the school and college students from the state university who serve full-time internships for one semester. The interns usually work in the school as classroom aides and provide tutoring and additional help to individual students. The residential staff members are college-educated men who are selected primarily on the basis of their ability to relate to the youngsters and to serve as adequate role models. Many of them are former college athletes who have expertise in supervising sports and other recreational activities. The teachers are selected on the basis of their ability to work well with students who have a history of poor achievement in school and behavior problems. Social services staff members have a master's degree in social work, counseling, or a related area. Outside consultants, including clinical psychologists, social workers, and other specialists, provide in-service training and additional supervision for staff and special services for residents, such as psychodrama, substance abuse workshops, career development workshops, and human sexuality groups.

GROUP LIVING

The group-living component provides direct residential supervision and recreational activities after school and on weekends. Specifically, group-living staff offer the residents structured experiences to help them learn, organize, and manage all the necessary skills for daily living, such as personal hygiene, laundry, meals (in the extension houses where residents do their own cooking), housework, and recreation. The basic tasks of the group-living staff are: (a) to serve as role models with regard to managing life challenges, such as handling anger, frustration, and interpersonal conflict; and (b) to monitor and supervise the functional demands of daily living. The residential staff members have the important task of creating a tone and psychological environment that is conducive to positive growth and change. The most important function of a group-living staff member is to form a relationship of mutual respect and trust with the residents and to help the residents develop the honesty and trust that is the basis for all meaningful and successful human relationships.

Philosophy of Group Living

The basic philosophy of the group-living department, as it is for the program as a whole, is that the development of a caring relationship is the prerequisite for successful treatment and rehabilitation. By forming strong relationships with the residents, the group-living staff can establish the trust that allows them to deal more effectively and openly with the residents' personal problems, peer relationships, and conflicts. In many ways, staff members try to provide the emotional support, structure, and role models that would be available in a healthy family environment.

The primary functional responsibilities of the group-living staff are to supervise daily activities, provide services such as transportation of residents to off-campus destinations, monitor interpersonal interactions among residents, supervise recreational activities, and be available for incidental and informal counseling on an as-needed basis. Specific tasks include coverage and supervision as designated by the senior staff person on duty, talking individually at least once a week to the boys assigned to the staff member's team, preparing team reports and attending team meetings, attending departmental staff meetings, and attending monthly meetings with the treatment director.

Careful, responsible, and consistent supervision is an essential function of the residential staff. Close supervision and consistent and fair discipline are the cornerstones that support successful treatment. Consistent confrontation on the "little things" often helps to establish a tone that is useful in dealing with larger problems when they occur.

Effective supervision involves acknowledging and rewarding positive behavior; setting appropriate limits on unacceptable behavior; and responding in a fair, reasonable, and consistent manner when residents overstep the boundaries. Effective supervision also requires the staff to ensure that the young men complete their functional tasks, such as keeping their rooms neat and clean, picking up after themselves, and doing assigned housework. It is interesting to note that of the 74% of the cases (n = 1,173) in the study for whom we have this information, most of the residents took good or excellent care of their rooms as reported in weekly progress reports from residential staff members. Specifically, 21.6% (n = 253) took excellent care; 63.2% took good care; and 6.2% (n = 73) were poor in keeping their rooms neat and clean. Another 9.6% (n = 106) were variable (response rate = 74%, n = 1,173). Residents not only take good care of their own rooms, but are also generally cooperative in completing other household chores: 23.8% (n = 298) "excellent"; 59.2% (n = 741) were "good"; 7.6% (n = 86) were "poor"; and 10% (n = 125) were "variable" (response rate = 79%, n = 1,252).

By demonstrating their ability to establish and maintain control in a firm, fair, and nonpunitive manner, the residential staff can create an environment in which the young men feel safe and protected. Although the residents may initially, and in some cases, continually challenge and rebel against the rules of the program and the residential staff's attempts to enforce them, in the long run, the residents are reassured by the staff's efforts to keep them out of trouble. In many ways, group-living staff members act as surrogate parents who care enough for their children to risk the unpopularity associated with setting limits and providing the required discipline.

Effective supervision involves more than providing discipline by sanctioning inappropriate behavior. It requires recognition and appreciation for positive behavior. It also requires flexibility, good judgment, knowing when to back off, coaxing, and a variety of other creative responses to deal with residents who at times can be volatile, unreasonable, and potentially dangerous. Effective supervision communicates to the residents the message: "I will do everything I can to help you stay out of further trouble because you have demonstrated that you are unable to control your behavior." Although a young man may initially rebel against this limit setting, the hope is that he ultimately finds it reassuring and comforting. The group-living staff has the challenge of not only making it clear to the residents that "the adults are in charge," but doing so in a manner that does not create an adversarial or "us against them" atmosphere.

The responsibilities of the group-living staff go far beyond routine supervision of daily tasks and maintaining orderly behavior. They are trying to assist the young men in the difficult and often frightening process of change. Providing the residents with an opportunity to change in a positive direction is the essential goal of the program. One of the most effective ways to help others learn how to act is to model the desired behavior. An important function of the residential staff is to provide role models for mature and socially acceptable behavior. All staff members have specific duties associated with their jobs. Their competence and creativity in implementing these responsibilities contribute significantly to their effectiveness. Equally important is their ability to relate to each other and to the residents in a professional and personally respectful manner. Role implementation is always carried out in the context of an interpersonal encounter. It is important for all staff to model through their own behavior how they expect the residents to act.

In general, the residents respond positively to the constructive and caring approach taken by residential staff members: 25% of the boys (n = 377) were "very cooperative with residential staff overall"; 57.8% (n = 847) were "moderately cooperative"; and 16.7% (n = 243) were "uncooperative" (response rate = 92.6%, n = 1,467).

Coverage of a Typical Day's Activities

Coverage involves the specific responsibilities of supervising the residents during the daytime, evening, and overnight shifts. Typically, coverage is provided by three-person shifts with a senior staff member in charge after school and in the evenings (3 p.m. to 11 p.m.) and by one person during the day (8 a.m. to 3 p.m.) and three staff members overnight (11 p.m. to 9:30 a.m.), two in the downstairs dormitory area and one upstairs in the smaller "honor" dormitory. The senior staff member assigns the specific responsibilities during a shift. On weekends, two staff members work shifts from 8 a.m. to 11 p.m. on Saturday and Sunday providing supervision for those residents who have either lost weekend-pass privileges or who are on the "new boy" (orientation) status. New residents do not receive weekend passes until they have successfully completed 5 weeks in the program.

Beginning with waking up at 7:30 a.m., group-living staff members are responsible for supervising all activities before breakfast, such as taking showers and making beds. At breakfast, staff members supervise the distribution of food (residents rotate the responsibility of serving the food) and remain in the dining room. After breakfast, they oversee any necessary housework until school begins at 9:30 a.m. During the school day, one residential staff member is responsible for general coverage and is assigned to the principal for any required errands or any other activity that is needed. Typical supervisory responsibilities during the school day include covering the dormitory area; handling the needs of sick residents (such as communicating to the teachers that a youngster is ill); dispensing medication; obtaining schoolwork from the teachers if the resident is unable to do it himself; supervising residents "on break" from classes; supervising boys who have been removed from class; coordinating out-of-class appointments; working with the residents assigned to setting up and serving lunch; assisting the teachers in supervising lunch; distributing mail during lunch; communicating relevant information to the staff members who are beginning coverage as the school day ends; and working on any special projects as assigned by the principal or director of group living.

After school, the residential staff members conduct and supervise an outdoor recreation program (weather permitting). This typically involves playing a seasonal sport and is mandatory for all residents unless they are too sick to participate. If youngsters cannot participate in recreation, one staff member stays with them. At 6 p.m., all the residents meet in the TV lounge for a brief meeting with the group-living staff to discuss any problems that may have arisen during the day. Residential staff members also supervise dinner.

Evening coverage begins after dinner. The senior staff member on duty assigns coverage for the evening. Usually, one staff member monitors the TV lounge, another staff member covers the gym, and a third staff member "floats." This last staff member is responsible for monitoring assigned housework and/or other sanctions. This is the most important time of the day in terms of the staff's interactions with the residents. Because there is less structured activity for the entire group at this time, there is a greater opportunity for increased negative behavior, such as teasing and fighting, fooling around, theft, illicit smoking or drug use, and so on. It is also the most opportune time for talking to the residents individually and providing incidental counseling.

Timing is one of the keys to effective intervention. As anyone who has ever worked in a mental hospital knows, patients often benefit as much or more from a conversation with a nurse or residential mental health worker who is available to the patient at the moment he or she wants to talk than they might from a weekly appointment with a psychiatrist, psychologist, or social worker. As the residential staff members are with the adolescents from the ending of school until bedtime, they are often in the best position to provide counsel to the adolescents when issues come up. Talking to a resident in private, whether in his room or in a car on the way to an appointment, can produce significant benefits in terms of the adolescent's behavior and his willingness to invest in the rehabilitation process. Although privacy is often essential for personal counseling and discussion, a staff member is never completely alone with the boy he is counseling. If the discussion is taking place in the adolescent's room, the door remains open. In other locations, the residential staff member and the resident are where others can see them.

The specific responsibilities of residential staff members during the evening shift include supervising the TV lounge, snack room, laundry, gym, and areas where the youngsters are likely to congregate; supervising showers between 9 p.m. and 10 p.m.; getting snacks after showers and returning them to the kitchen; periodically checking the cleanliness of the TV lounge and snack room; ensuring that these rooms are clean and in order by 11 p.m.; making sure that no one enters the dormitory area except to take a shower; finding time to have individual and small group discussions and counseling with the residents; and keeping in close communication with other staff on duty. In general, it is important for the staff to (a) keep moving and not stay in one area; (b) be sensitive to the mood of the group as well as particular individuals and to communicate this to other staff; and (c) to communicate any problems to other staff.

Night coverage is the responsibility of two staff members from 11 p.m. to 9:30 a.m. This staff member has a number of duties. These include checking the residents every 30 minutes from 11 p.m. until 1 a.m. and every hour after that; to shut off the residents' radios at midnight; to check on the cleanliness of the building, noting and recording any damage on the night coverage form; checking and recording supplies (i.e., housework cleaning supplies and snacks) that need to be ordered; repairing vacuum cleaners and other equipment; giving out and recording prescribed medications; communicating "significant behaviors" to the next shift on the night coverage form; waking the boys and assisting with breakfast; assisting with supervision during housework; and being familiar with each young man's treatment goals and special needs, particularly those that may apply at night, such as waking up residents with a history of wetting their beds, recording nightmares, and so on.

The group-living staff members have an important, difficult, and emotionally demanding job. Adolescents who end up in residential placement typically have difficulty with self-discipline, accepting responsibility, completing assigned tasks, and listening to authority. When confronted with responsibility, demands, rules, structure, frustration, or other practical or psychological demands, these youngsters often respond poorly. They are likely to be noncooperative, hostile, verbally and occasionally physically abusive, manipulative, and/or overreactive in their responses. Basically, the residential staff member is in the role of a surrogate parent with youngsters who often have a history of insufficient, ineffective, neglectful, or abusive parenting. These youngsters may have learned to constantly challenge and resist authority, even when it is nurturing and caring. It is no simple task to raise a family of 30 or more kids, all of whom are teenagers!

FORMAL EDUCATION

The Ocean Tides School is certified by the state department of education for grades 7 through 12 and is fully accredited by the NEASC. The school program allows the youngster to continue his education while in placement and, in some cases, after placement is completed. As many of the residents have fallen behind their appropriate grade level because of past failures and poor performance in school, the school program is structured to allow some residents to make accelerated progress by taking double credits. In this way, a young man can complete two school years in one. This is particularly important for remotivating residents who may have given up because of past failures. Regardless of intelligence or other abilities, many of the residents may have adopted negative attitudes toward school and have evolved an attitude of "learned helplessness" because they are so far behind. A major goal of the school is not only to educate these young men but also to help them change their attitudes toward school, their capacity to learn, and their potential for success. The guiding principle is if the youngsters feel that their teachers care about them and there is trust in their relationship with their teachers, they will change their beliefs about their ability to learn. They will now think that they can learn, even though they did not previously think they could.

In addition to a standardized curriculum, the Ocean Tides School employs several innovative techniques to teach these youngsters, many of whom have special needs. The teachers establish individual educational goals for each child that are realistic and allow for successful goal attainment. Tutoring, remedial work, and the creation of special learning projects of particular interest to the students supplement their regular classroom instruction. Classes are small and students can work at their own pace. Students receive individual attention and their progress is carefully monitored. The school's goal is to break the pattern of failure experienced by these young men in their prior educational experiences and to instill self-motivation and a desire to learn. These goals cannot be achieved without dedicated and compassionate teachers and the program emphasizes the establishment of a strong relationship between teacher and student. As Lindner and Wagner (1983, p. 28) commented: "The teacher is not seen merely as a provider of knowledge, but as a motivating force for educational growth. Educational staff are selected not only on the basis of their teaching abilities, but because they are warm, supportive persons."

Educational Philosophy

The philosophy of the Ocean Tides School is consistent with the previously described program philosophy that incorporates aspects of Reality Therapy and LaSallian principles. The school operates under the assumption that knowledge and wisdom are most likely to occur in a context of enthusiastic inquiry. Much knowledge can be gained though the experience of living and without formal study of education. Many of the residents at Ocean Tides have demonstrated this by indicating considerable levels of "street smarts" despite undistinguished academic records. As an institution of learning, a school has the responsibility and goal of organizing personnel, space, time, materials, and curriculum so that knowledge can be made more accessible. The Ocean Tides School is dedicated to the intelligent search for knowledge through creative exploration. It is based on the belief that a school both furnishes the tools necessary for inquiry and indicates paths of investigation that can bring students to greater knowledge of themselves, their abilities, the world in which they live, and the traditions and cultures of human society. In so doing, the school provides an education that encourages the students to understand their personal, communal, and cultural past. The school attempts to provide the students with the ability to analyze the present and plan for the future.

Ocean Tides does not presume that the adolescents entering the school program are students who are eager to learn or enthusiastic about attending class. On the contrary, the school program recognizes that many of the youngsters have a history of school failure and truancy and may have developed negative attitudes toward school. The school attempts to avoid potentially negative consequences of giving up on the adolescent and accepting a self-fulfilling prophecy of failure and setting unrealistic and unreachable goals that invite failure. The challenge is to move the young men from ennui, self-doubt, and negative attitudes toward learning to the systemic search for knowledge and self-improvement. To accomplish this, the Ocean Tides School (a) uses a careful diagnostic and prescriptive procedure that is individually tailored to each student; (b) has a variety of curriculum offerings; and (c) utilizes a "building blocks" approach to curriculum organization that allows each student the opportunity to make real and discernible progress. The teaching approach recognizes that the search for knowledge is affected by the formal curriculum, the informal tone of the school, and the attitudes of the teachers. The school values fairness, openness, humor, cooperation, honesty, curiosity, creativity, and self-esteem. The fundamental belief is that students can recognize whether or not the school cares about them and that learning occurs most successfully in a context of caring.

Educational Goals

The Ocean Tides School distinguishes between two interrelated types of goals: program goals, which are the educational aspirations for the school itself, and inquiry goals, which are the objectives for the students. The program goals are: (a) that the school works in harmony with the residential program for the maximum benefit of the residents;

(b) that each student's program offers real opportunity for success and challenge; (c) that the school plans each student's program on an individual basis; (d) that the school helps students develop individual and social responsibility; and (e) that the school draws upon the residential–community experience of the students as an area of inquiry and education by using group-living experiences in life management, money management, group trips, volunteering in the community, and other comparable experiences as a basis for education.

Inquiry goals for students are developed in detail in connection with each curriculum block. General guidelines include the following: (a) that students increase their desire to know more, their willingness to study, and their ability to work more systematically; (b) that students develop and improve basic skills, including the ability to read with comprehension, to write with clarity, to compute with accuracy, and to listen attentively; (c) that students develop an understanding of human history and of political and social institutions; (d) that students develop an appreciation for beauty; (e) that students develop some understanding of the physical universe and of life systems; and (f) that students learn skills and interests that give them feelings of satisfaction, enjoyment, and accomplishment that help to bring about order in their lives.

School Programming

In order to realize a positive and successful school experience for each boy, the school program has been designed to allow for flexible scheduling, highly individualized program planning, small student–teacher ratios, and careful monitoring of each youngster's progress. The school program is organized around the major academic disciplines, with enrichment curricula in the areas of personal development. Each student participates in English, mathematics, social studies, science, industrial arts, and physical education. In addition, each boy participates in a series of 8-week courses in areas of personal development that include art, culinary arts, horticulture, woodworking, wood turning, and human "survival skills" (health, human sexuality, drug use and awareness, and skills for independent living). There is an opportunity for special classes and programs as described later in the chapter.

School Calendar

As mandated by the Rhode Island state law, the school year consists of 180 days and is divided into four quarters of approximately 8 weeks each. In addition, there is a 7-week summer school session that most students attend. At the end of each quarter, there is a Reflection Day, a special day that is set aside to afford students and staff the opportunity to reflect on the completed cycles. The Reflection Day allows the young men an opportunity to assess their participation in the school program over the past quarter. This is a time when the residents are encouraged to recognize their achievement (or lack of them) and to set new goals for the next quarter. Each reflection day includes a formal award ceremony in which each youngster receives a certificate indicating the academic credits he has earned and acknowledging any additional individual achievement, accomplishments, and progress in the program. In addition, certificates are awarded for particular accomplishments, such as most improved, least sanctions, and so on. Frequently, Reflection Days incorporate a specific theme or focus on an upcoming holiday. A special celebration meal, such as a banquet or special breakfast, is usually included in the Reflection Day activities.

School Orientation

When a young man is accepted into the program, the principal meets with the teachers to summarize pertinent information from prior school experiences and to inform the staff when the student will begin classes. On arrival, the school orientation program consists of the following activities: a staff member is assigned to the student to describe the school program, help him complete the New Student Inventory Form, and review the student handbook. The student signs a statement agreeing to participate in the school program. This process usually takes 1 day to complete. When the various aspects of the orientation process have been completed, the principal and teachers meet to review test results and other material and to make up a class schedule. During the first few weeks of the resident's participation in school, there will be ongoing discussion to determine and shape the educational plan for the young man. During this time period, Ocean Tides will request transcripts and other pertinent data from the resident's prior schools. The youngster's progress is reviewed after 1 month. An individual educational plan (IEP) and subject area plans by each teacher will be prepared after 45 days.

Student Evaluation

Each student's school participation and progress is monitored closely. *Daily sheets* are used as feedback from staff to students. At the end of each day, the teaching staff adds a comment on the progress of the student in school. The statement is short and constructive. Students can read these comments the following morning during homeroom. The *point sheet* is a comprehensive assessment of the student's progress throughout the school program. New point sheets are distributed on Monday morning in homeroom. The sheet has a numerical value each day ranging from 0 to 5 in certain classroom requirements, such as appropriate behavior, classwork, cooperation, language, and respect. The boy receives one point for each completed requirement. A zero in class work will result in time taken off the boy's weekend pass. *Learner outcomes* are statements of what student should know and be able to accomplish by the end of each quarter. They are based on the curriculum for each course the student takes. The learner outcome form begins with a summary of what the course is designed to accomplish.

The school expects each student to achieve his learner outcomes with a certain percent of mastery depending on the individual student's abilities. Every student has a set of learner outcomes for each course. These help him and the teacher stay focused on what needs to be taught and learned during the quarter. Learner outcomes are due by the end of the second week of each quarter. *Treatment notes* are a monthly obligation for all teachers. They give an overall outline of the boy's progress in school. Overall behavior as well as how a young man is doing academically are discussed. The treatment notes describe staff and peer interactions and suggest goals for the month. Each teacher has the responsibility of writing a short progress summary for several students. The *advisory program* is a structured time during which special activities are designed and implemented to help students fulfill their identified needs with consistent, caring, and continuous guidance. Finally, each teacher is responsible for maintaining a *portfolio* that consists of a working folder and a digital portfolio of the student's work. The working folder is a compilation of the student's corrected work. Every 1 or 2 weeks, the student is encouraged to select something from his working folder that shows what he has learned. He writes a few lines stating why he chose that piece of work to go into his portfolio. Contents of a possible portfolio may contain a journal entry, a photograph of a project, tests, reports, videotapes, audiotapes, art activities, graphs, charts, teacher observations, and cooperative group events.

Daily School Procedures

The teachers arrive at 8:45 a.m. and begin each day with a 30-minute meeting. The purpose of this meeting is to facilitate communication among the staff and is used for planning, announcements, and dealing with individual issues. At each Friday's morning meeting, the clinical psychologist meets with the teachers to discuss any issues and to summarize his most recent assessment of one of the residents. There is an informational meeting with the residents scheduled on Thursday afternoons to announce plans for the following week and to address any general issues. The residents and teachers all meet together at 9:25 a.m. and the teachers take the students in their respective classes to begin the school day. The school day goes from 9:30 a.m. until 3:30 p.m. and is divided into class periods of 45 minutes. The school follows a rotating schedule so that different classes meet at different times on each day. Makeup work and sanctions can be completed between 3 p.m. and 3:30 p.m.

Role of the Teacher

Teaching at Ocean Tides is a demanding and challenging task. Many if not most of the residents have a history of problems in school, including poor academic performance, behavior problems, low motivation, and truancy. The information in Table 5.1 illustrates the past academic behavior and motivational histories of the residents.

Because of their past problems in school, the residents often arrive with strong negative feelings toward school and teachers. It is essential that teachers have the personal qualities and professional skills to counter the negative attitudes that have developed through repeated failure,

TABLE 5.1
Past Academic Behavior and Motivation

	ACADEMIC SUCCESS (n = 1,464, 92.4%)	BEHAVIOR IN SCHOOL (n = 1,409, 88.9%)	MOTIVATION IN SCHOOL (n = 1,413, 89.1%)
Consistently poor	741 (46.8)	795 (50.2)	885 (55.8)
Consistently average	235 (14.8)	225 (14.2)	185 (11.7)
Consistently above average	60 (3.8)	40 (2.5)	33 (2.1)
Variable	176 (11.1)	127 (8.0)	126 (7.9)
Variable, ranging from average–poor to poor–average	252 (15.9)	222 (14.0)	184 (11.6)

Note: Simple Pearson's coefficient calculations are all statistically significant at the .01 level indicating that estimates of the extent to which responses across all three items are similar are as predicted: For example, boys who performed poorly in academics tended also to behave poorly and were poorly motivated in school. Counts are raw numbers and percents are in parentheses.

confrontation with teachers, and disciplinary action. Successful teaching and learning are most likely to occur in a context of mutual trust and respect. In order to facilitate the development of this trust, perhaps for the first time, it is essential that the teachers at Ocean Tides (a) encourage and support students in ways that will allow them to begin to dispel their fear of failure; (b) provide experiences of success to counter the young men's prior negative experiences in school; (c) instruct and make demands in a manner that is caring and consistent so that learning can take place; and (d) set limits so that poor behavior does not prevent or interfere with learning.

Teachers engage in the traditional activities, such as classroom instruction, curriculum development, long-range planning, and immediate preparation. However, the role of the teacher in the Ocean Tides School goes beyond the traditional roles of the classroom teacher. The teacher contributes to the total rehabilitation of the youngsters. This requires effective communication skills, personal initiative, interpersonal sensitivity, and the ability to remain calm in dealing with sudden, unprovoked, verbally aggressive, or similar difficult behavior. In addition to being responsible for innovative and highly individualized teaching in the classroom, the teacher participates as a member of a treatment team for several youngsters and supervises residents outside of the classroom, such as lunchtime. Teachers are responsible for keeping clear and accurate records of course attendance and credits; monitoring individual behavior by completing Daily Lifestyle

Sheets, Review Reports, IEPs and incident reports. Finally, the teacher is available for "incidental" counseling that may be initiated "spontaneously" by a resident. In many ways, the teacher at Ocean Tides is more accurately described as an educational therapist. In general, interactions between teachers and residents are positive: 27.1% (n = 429) of the boys are "very cooperative" with teachers, 52.7% (n = 835) are "moderately cooperative," and only 10.6% (n = 166) are "uncooperative" (response rate = 90.2%, n = 1,430).

Role of the Principal

The principal assumes responsibility for ensuring that the educational component of the program is in compliance with all state and federal regulations and accreditation criteria so that the school maintains its status as licensed and accredited. In view of the often severe educational problems that the young men have experienced in the past, it is the principal's responsibility to ensure that a creative and individualized educational program is established for each resident and that this educational plan conforms to the goals and objectives of his total treatment plan. The principal has the task and responsibility for administering all aspects of the school, including instructional management; monitoring and maintaining school improvement; managing personnel; management of fiscal, administrative, and facilities functions; student management; community relations; and professional growth and development. Some of the more important specific responsibilities include (a) attending monthly administrative treatment meetings and presenting progress reports on each youngster, providing specific recommendations regarding the educational needs of each youngster, and giving input regarding the ability of the department to implement the approved goals and objectives; (b) working with the administration in establishing a system for the delivery of educational services consistent with state and federal regulations and the philosophy and goals of the program; (c) assuming responsibility for the direct supervision and professional growth of the educational staff, including formal evaluations of each teacher; (d) working with the president on budgeting and financial needs for the school; (e) being familiar with current treatment trends in juvenile delinquency and child care and ensure that the educational component incorporates and reflects these trends; and (f) representing the school at the variety of meetings and conferences involved with treating the residents. In brief, the principal has the authority and responsibility to implement and supervise all the specific activities related to the education of the young men in the program.

Role of the Assistant Principal

The assistant principal is in charge of the Providence Campus of Ocean Tides School and reports to the principal. The assistant principal's duties and responsibilities include instructional management (participating in the development and evaluation of the education program, supporting development of innovative instructional programs by teachers, and promoting the use of technology for teachers and students); managing school–organizational climate (promoting a positive, caring climate for learning; dealing sensitively and fairly with persons from diverse cultural, ethnic, and racial backgrounds; and communicating effectively with students and staff); school–organizational improvement; assisting the principal with personnel management; administration of the Providence Campus (including fiscal and facilities management); student management (ensuring adequate supervision of students, maintaining an effective discipline system that results in positive student behavior, and conducting conferences on student and school issues with parents, students, and teachers); and participating in professional growth and development.

Role of the Director of Special Education

The director has the legal responsibility to affect and maintain compliance with federal and state education regulations and laws as they pertain to the students and their families. The director is the administrator for both campuses of Ocean Tides School appointed to interview and enroll new students referred by the local educational agency (LEA) special education directors and is the liaison between Ocean Tides and the public schools. The essential duties and responsibilities of the special education director are to track all IEP due dates so that each IEP is written in a timely manner at both campuses; be the primary resource for all teachers to keep them informed of changes in the special education regulations, processes, and procedures; remain current on all general education regulations to ensure any and all changes in graduation requirement are implemented; actively seek to increase enrollment at both campuses of special education students; with the principal, advocate for change to improve the educational experience of all students; maintain positive relationships and network with directors of special education in the state; and complete the yearly special education application and the Individuals With Disabilities Education Act part of the Consolidated Resource Plan.

Role of the Guidance Counselor–Work/Study Coordinator

This important position has a number of responsibilities related to the vocational program and postsecondary education. The specific duties include planning and implementation of the special days (Career Day at the Providence Campus, Substance Abuse Day, Sexuality Awareness Day, Vocational Assessments at the Providence Campus); employment counseling for students not planning to attend college; helping seniors at both campuses complete financial aid forms; investigating postsecondary options; applications to colleges for seniors at both campuses; applications to vocational schools and other career–technology centers; applications to private high schools; counseling for nonresidential students; facilitating return to public high schools for students leaving the program; overseeing state testing at both campuses; setting up Scholastic Aptitude Tests at both campuses; and monitoring the process of job procurement and employment by students.

Special Classes and Programs

Art Class

The art class involves the students in a variety of projects designed to activate their imagination, creativity, and problem solving. The students' art training is integrated with their community service. For example, they have an annual sale of ceramic bowls that they have made and the proceeds go to support the Rhode Island Food Bank. Among the projects they create are clay murals to which all of the residents contribute; plaster and clay masks; mosaics made from glass and mixed materials;

and painted murals on the walls of both school campuses. The students receive instruction in basic drawing and learn about art history. An exhibition of their paintings and drawings has been displayed at the local hospital.

Culinary Arts Program

The culinary arts program at Ocean Tides School began in 1992. Chef Andy Lussier, an experienced chef, teacher, faculty member, and executive chef at the Johnson and Wales University School of Culinary Arts was hired initially as a consultant and then as a full-time teacher to develop and administer a culinary arts program. This program is part of the total education program at Ocean Tides and consists of both instruction periods and "hands on" experiences. The students are instructed in baking; cold food preparation; making of sauces, soups, and entrees; knife skills; how to take inventory; and proper sanitation. Phase I of the program lasts 5 weeks and involves five students. Phase II is a more advanced course and the top five students from the three Phase I programs are chosen for this course. During Phase I, the boys are responsible for the lunch service for the other students and help prepare the dinner meal. They are taught how to set a table and serve a meal. When special functions take place, they are involved as professional waiters and learn the fine points of serving a meal. There is a special class after school where the students learn how to plan a menu, shop for the food, prepare the food, and serve it to a group of students and staff members. They go to the extension houses and put on a dinner for the residents. With the experience at Ocean Tides, many of the students get jobs in the local restaurants, especially during the summer. While Chef Lussier is the main teacher, two other chefs assist him. At the Providence Campus, there is a program in food preparation that includes instruction and practice in basic cooking, food safety, and cleanliness. The students prepare the lunch meal under the supervision of a trained cook.

Horticulture Class

The horticulture class is a one-semester course consisting of academic training and practical experience. Topics include types of soil and how plants use soil; plant biology; how to prepare, plant, and clean out a garden; greenhouse planning and how to use a greenhouse; aquaculture;

types of pesticides and pesticide safety; organic controls; irrigation and watering systems; pests; diseases; parasites; crop rotation; and other relevant topics. The students do field work in which they gather soil samples, identify plant species; and plant both a fall and spring vegetable garden. The vegetables are used for a spring plant sale and also in the culinary program for food preparation.

Wood-Turning Class

The wood-turning class is designed to increase the students' feelings of self-esteem, pride, and self-confidence by teaching them how to make a variety of practical objects using a lathe and corresponding tools. The class is structured for students to gradually advance from beginner projects to more advanced projects. There are four phases. In Phase I, the students make practical objects they can bring home to their families. These include spatulas, bottle stoppers, and pens. In Phase II, the students learn to make simple round boxes. Phase III involves learning the more complex constructions of bowls. Phase IV is the most advanced stage and the process is opened up for students to make whatever they want. Some of the projects made in this phase are stools, small chairs, and small tables.

Woodworking Class

The students begin class with constructing a hat and coat rack. This project introduces the students to a variety of skills needed in woodworking, such as the proper use of power tools, how to drill, measurement and layout, and finishing (sanding, staining, and applying the finish). From this project, students move on to making a basic box, which involves learning how to join. Students can individualize their boxes and this helps create and maintain their interest. For example, one student made a heart-shaped box as a present for his girlfriend in which her smartphone could be kept. Students learn how to use wood burning for decorating their projects. The residents have built a wide variety of objects, including a replica of an antique rocking horse, kitchen trivets and serving trays, and small bureaus and tables. Some of the objects created in the woodshop have been used as door prize, raffle, or auction items to raise money for charity. Some of the tools that the students learn to use are a table saw, band saw, jigsaw, compound miter saw, drill press, router and router cables, sanders, and wood-burning tools.

Vocational Programs

Vocational training programs are available at both campuses of Ocean Tides School. These programs include workshops and classes in plumbing, electrical wiring, landscape architecture, and carpentry or woodworking. Master craftsmen who have been hired as adjunct faculty teach in these workshops and classes. In addition to teaching the basic skills, the teachers provide valuable information about a career in the respective occupations. They indicate the type of training and certification required in the short- and long-term compensation, and the difficult aspects of the job. Students get the opportunity for practical application of the skills under the supervision of the teachers. For example, one of the projects at the Providence Campus involved the construction of a greenhouse. The students put the greenhouse shell together on a lot adjacent to the school; dug trenches to contain the plumbing and wiring from the school to the greenhouse; connected the pipes and wires needed; installed the heating, fan, and lighting systems; and built the necessary benches and shelves. After the greenhouse was completed, the students landscaped the outside and installed planting beds under the guidance of the consulting landscape architect.

The most extensive vocational program is the building maintenance or construction class. Working with the master carpenter or cabinet maker, the students converted the double garage belonging to one of the former group homes into a state-of-the-art woodworking and carpentry shop. They used this facility to build the cabinets and counters for a remodeled and modern kitchen in the group home that is used for the food preparation program. The vocational instruction is divided between traditional classroom instruction and hands-on community-based projects. Students use the community as their laboratory where all projects are real-life experiences of helping those in need. Students have the opportunity to earn an Occupational Safety and Health Administration (OSHA) certification card necessary for work in the trades.

Teacher Evaluations

The evaluation process is designed to provide an ongoing, structured forum within which discussion, observation, and evaluation of staff performance may be addressed. The process is intended to allow staff members the opportunity to reflect on their work, receive feedback, identify areas of need, recognize areas of demonstrated strengths, encourage the teachers' continuing professional development, and provide the school with an additional basis for improvement and program development. The specific format for teacher evaluation is as follows. The principal formally observes each teacher at least twice during the school year. Following the class observation, the teacher and principal meet to go over how the teacher views his or her work and to discuss the observation. Following this discussion, the principal prepares a written evaluation that includes a summary of the evaluation, point of commendation, and recommendations. The teacher has the option of attaching a self-evaluation or other comments relative to the written evaluation. The principal and teacher have a follow-up meeting to discuss the written evaluation and plan strategies for implementing any recommendations. The signed copy of the written evaluation is included in the teacher's personnel file.

SOCIAL SERVICES AND COUNSELING

Social Services Department

The social services department is responsible for providing individual and family counseling services and other support services to the residents and their families. A major goal of the Ocean Tides program is to successfully reunite each adolescent with his family. The social services counselors establish regular contact with the youngsters and their families and attempt to bridge the gap between the families and the young men in residence. Each counselor is assigned to youngsters and has the responsibility of implementing a prescriptive treatment program that has been specifically designed for each resident and his family. This treatment plan includes individual counseling for the resident, family counseling for the resident and relevant family members, home visits, and any other services that are required. One of the unique and most effective aspects of the Ocean Tides program has been the provision of regular family counseling throughout the duration of the resident's stay in the program. This is important because of the three types of rehabilitation programs that have been found to be effective through rigorous scientific evaluation and empirical validation; two of them (functional family therapy and multisystem family therapy) involve family counseling (Guerra, Kim, & Boxer, 2008). Ocean Tides has been working with the adolescents and their families almost since its inception and was one of the first programs in the country to incorporate family counseling as a regular and essential feature of its treatment.

Social Services Goals

The social services department has individual and family counseling as its main focus with the ultimate goal of providing enough change in the family system to facilitate successful reintegration of the adolescent with his family when he completes the program. Specific departmental goals include helping the young man to gain a fuller realization of his strengths and abilities; attempting to resolve existing conflicts and problems that interfere with his ability to cope with family, peers, authority, and the community; and developing realistic goals that can be achieved once the resident has completed the program and returned home. In working with the families, the goals include improving communication; establishing a realistic system of family rules and sanctions; helping each family member to learn more effective and positive ways of interacting; and giving support and positive reinforcement to the parent(s) in their role as executive(s) of the family.

Social Services Staff

The staff, including the department director, consists of three men and three women. Five of the six staff members have their master's degree in either clinical social work or marital and family therapy and are licensed by the state for the independent practice of psychotherapy or counseling. One staff member is fluent in Spanish and can work with those families where neither parent speaks English. All of them have years of experience working with delinquent male adolescents.

Role of the Director of Social Services

The director of the social services department administers the department and is responsible for establishing programs consistent with the philosophy and goals of the Ocean Tides program. Specific duties include presenting progress reports on each resident and his family at the monthly meetings of the administrative team; making specific recommendations regarding the treatment needs of each adolescent and his family; giving specific feedback about the ability of the social services department to implement its programs and achieve its goals; providing case supervision for the social services staff; establishing and carrying out a system for input into the court letters documenting a resident's progress (or lack thereof), treatment meetings, case conferences, and other treatment planning activities; handling all administrative tasks within the department, such as hiring, firing, scheduling, evaluation of staff, accreditation reports, and so on; and sharing on-call responsibilities with the other administrators. The director is both an administrator and clinician who provides both leadership and an exemplary professional role model for the social services staff.

Social Services Counselor

The responsibilities of the social services counselor are to implement the specific treatment goals that have been developed for a particular resident and his family that have been approved by the administrative team. These goals are listed in the written ITP that is placed in the resident's case file. In general, these responsibilities involve development and maintenance of a therapeutic relationship with each resident and his family; regular and consistent individual and family counseling sessions; participation in selected group counseling programs; providing information to the families concerning available community resources; monitoring all weekend passes and other home-visit activities through the weekend sheets that are completed by the parents; phone contacts and home visits with parents and other relevant family members; and maintenance of regular contact with other agencies involved with the young man, such as probation, drug treatment, and so on.

Individual and family counseling is an important function of the social services staff. As the following data indicate, cooperation by both the resident and his family is variable: 77% ($n = 1{,}220$) of the boys had at least one relative who was either "moderately" or "very" cooperative with counseling services, and 90.8% of the boys themselves were either "moderately" or "very" cooperative with counseling services.

In addition to the provision of direct services, social services staff members participate in all scheduled department and other staff meetings, direct supervision with the department director and/or his designee (e.g., an outside consultant), and in workshops and other training opportunities both within and outside of the agency. Social services staff members are accountable for keeping accurate and up-to-date records of all counseling and intervention activities and for providing regular written reports and summaries of their interventions and interactions. The social services staff members are expected to possess strong skills in interpersonal communication, personal initiative, empathy, a caring attitude, and sensitivity. They are encouraged to maintain these qualities through ongoing supervision, in-service training, and continuing professional education.

Individual Counseling

All of the residents have regularly scheduled weekly counseling sessions with their assigned social services counselor. Adolescence is a difficult developmental stage. Normal issues, such as gender identity, body image, peer pressure to experiment with drugs and alcohol, and emerging needs to establish one's individual identity and separate from family, all contribute to the adolescent's need to talk things over with someone who is trusted and respected. In addition to the normal developmental issues associated with adolescence, our residents usually have additional stressors resulting from chaotic and unstable family situations, gang-related conflict, premature fatherhood, trouble with the police, and failure in school. In other words, they have a lot to be talked about.

Although the adolescents in the program need counseling, they are often not good candidates for traditional counseling because they lack insight and are not psychologically minded. In the novel *Moonlight Mile* (Lehane, 2010), there is a conversation between a detective and a social worker about an adolescent girl who has gotten into trouble with the law. The detective tells the social worker that he cannot get a clear picture of the youngster and the social worker explains that is because a clear picture does not exist. She goes on to say that the girl entered adolescence with "no real skills, no ambition, and zero sense of self. She's smart enough to know she has deficiencies but not smart enough to know what they are…Sophie's what I call a floater. She bobs along waiting for someone to come along and tell her where to go" (Lehane, 2010, p. 150).

Although the foregoing description is that of an adolescent female rather than a male, it accurately depicts many of our young men who are not amenable to counseling, so traditional counseling techniques are difficult to use and doomed to failure. More success can be achieved by more informal and "incidental" counseling that occurs on an "as-needed" basis. In addition to the regularly scheduled formal counseling sessions provided by each resident's social worker, residential staff members provide ongoing "incidental" counseling.

Prior to coming to Ocean Tides, many or even most of our residents have received little, if any, positive attention from adults. Sometimes this is because the adolescents have not engaged in much behavior that is deserving of praise or positive attention. However, even when they have demonstrated positive behavior, it has often gone unnoticed and unrewarded. As a result, many of the adolescents who come into the program have serious and chronically low levels of self-esteem. At a core level, they do not believe that they deserve to be successful. The following anecdote provides a good example of this negative belief system. One of the residents who had completed the program was continuing his high school education at the Providence Campus of Ocean Tides School. However, his attendance had dropped off and he was in jeopardy of being dropped. He claimed that he had no way of getting to school because he could not get a bus pass and no one in his family could give him a ride. When one of the teachers offered to pick him up on his way to school, the student replied: "You would do that for me!"

Although modern society puts great emphasis on the importance of self-esteem and feeling good about oneself, there is less clarity about how to develop a positive self-image. Self-esteem develops from competence, actual achievements, and mastery of the skills necessary for social survival. Although high achievement is no guarantee of positive self-esteem, true self-esteem is earned and reality based. The paradox of self-esteem is that in order to acquire it, one needs to have mastered certain skills. However, a certain amount of self-esteem is required to have the confidence to try and learn those skills.

Because of past negative experiences, many of our residents are both hesitant and reluctant to trust adults enough to open up. Therefore, it is important that staff notice positive behavior and reward it by providing positive feedback. Even when staff members try to be open, empathic, and helpful, the residents will resist their best efforts. It is important for staff not to become discouraged when their initial attempts to establish a positive relationship fail. The challenge for the counselor is to overcome the resistance. Trust, like respect, must be earned. It is advisable to proceed with caution and allow the adolescent sufficient time to discover that the staff member can be trusted. For the staff member, the key is to be available and to be a good listener. Close and attentive listening is often all that is needed. Most important of all, the counselor is genuine, truthful, and honest. Although residents may not excel in the classroom, they are "street smart" and interpersonally savvy. They can sense a phony and often can tell if someone is being patronizing or gratuitous.

Family Counseling

Working with the families of the residents is an important and integral part of the treatment program and is conducted by the social services staff. The social services counselors work primarily on trying to help the family remove existing barriers to communication, diminish the amount of anger in the family and replace it with more positive feelings, help the parent(s) establish appropriate structure and discipline, and clarify family roles. Family meetings are conducted either weekly or biweekly either in a location convenient for the family or in the family home. When the group homes were still open, these provided accessible sites because of their locations in different parts of the state. As the group homes have closed, the Providence Campus of Ocean Tides School has become the meeting place of choice after the school has closed. If the resident is involved in the family meeting, a staff member transports him to the meeting location. Home visits in the evenings are common so that employed parents do not have to miss work.

Group Therapy

Ocean Tides utilizes a variety of group therapy, counseling, and psychoeducational groups for the residents. The focus and frequency of the groups vary according to the needs of the specific group of residents in placement at a given time and the availability of qualified staff and consultants to conduct the groups. Typically, the groups are time limited, topic focused, and structured. Over the years, several types of group therapy have been offered, including milieu therapy groups, sexual offender treatment groups, new father groups (4.9%, $n = 78$ of the boys have biological children of their own), leadership, psychodrama, social skills training, substance abuse, and anger management. Some examples of types of groups and special programs that have been offered are described in the following sections.

Psychodrama

This group existed for many years but is not currently offered because the consultant who led the group is no longer available. The group met once per week for 8-week sequences throughout the school year and all residents in the program participated in the group on a rotated basis. The group leader was a consultant with expertise in psychodrama. Staff members had the opportunity to serve as participant observers. The group utilized psychodrama, role-playing, and other active group therapy techniques to explore common personal problems and conflicts.

An important aspect of rehabilitating delinquent young men is to provide them with the opportunity to increase their self-esteem by participating in noncriminal and socially redeeming activities. Often, delinquent youngsters have not had the opportunity to engage in the kinds of social activities that allow them to learn new skills and have positive experiences. Ocean Tides has developed a number of special activities to supplement and enhance the regular program.

Leadership Group

One of the most powerful influences on adolescent behavior is peer pressure. The leadership group was designed to use peer pressure to change negative, attention-getting behavior into more positive, socially proactive behavior. The leadership groups are intermittent because they are dependent on being able to identify students in the program with leadership potential. The group is a semi-structured psychoeducational group. The coleaders are the consultant in clinical psychology, the guidance/vocational counselor, and sometimes a third staff member, such as the director of residential living. The group runs for 6 weeks with no more than six participants. Two sessions are devoted to each of the three topics: defining leadership, communication skills and decision making, and problem solving. The first topic (defining leadership) involves brainstorming and trying to define the major components of leadership and the characteristics of a good or effective leader. The group leaders begin each phase with Socratic questioning of the participants to get their ideas before they are given information, skill training, or exercises. The following concepts and tasks are covered in the first phase: the difference between thoughts and feelings; how negative thoughts contribute to low self-esteem, common self-defeating beliefs (handout); and two self-esteem exercises. The second phase (communication skills) involves teaching how good communication skills are essential to effective leadership. Initial brainstorming includes asking what are good communication skills and the importance of being a good listener. The leaders distribute handouts on three characteristics of effective listening and good versus bad communication, including the difference between clear, direct, masked, and indirect communication patterns. After discussing the distributed material, the group uses role-playing techniques to practice the skills. The last phases, sessions 5 and 6, deal with how to make good decisions and solve problems. The leaders identify different stages in the problem-solving process, such as identifying the problem, communicating it to the appropriate person, developing different action strategies and deciding on an effective one, and evaluating the success or failure of the decision. The group applies these principles to specific problems using group discussion and dyadic role-plays.

Sexual Awareness Group

The sexual awareness group is an educational group conducted in the evening by one of the teachers for 6 weeks. Each session lasts 90 minutes. The topics discussed include reproduction facts, relationship issues, sexually transmitted diseases, and safe sex practices.

Substance Abuse Counseling

Staff members from Phoenix House, a substance abuse treatment program, provide substance abuse counseling both in a 12-week psychoeducational group format and also for selected individuals as needed.

Skill Development Groups

Because of their difficulties in peer relations and interpersonal relations in general, Ocean Tides developed social skills training groups. The social skills groups have a membership of six residents and focus on helping the young men learn to relate to each other more effectively. These groups are time-limited and semi-structured, using exercises and role-playing to increase skill development. The goals of the group are to increase social skills, listening skills, and communication skills.

Anger Management Group

This is an ongoing group that includes those young men with a documented history of aggressive behavior and poor impulse control with regard to anger. Depending on who is leading the group, a variety of formats have been used over the years. These range from highly structured groups utilizing video modeling and role-playing format, to less structured approaches that rely primarily on group discussion. In addition to the group format, one of the consultant clinical psychologists does anger management training with individual students on a weekly basis. These individual sessions last from an hour to an hour and a half.

One approach that was used for several years was a program developed by Dr. Rodney Hammond (Hammond & Yung, 1991) called "Givin' It, Takin' It, and 'Workin' It Out." This was a video-based program that illustrated through the use of before-and-after scenes how conflict can be managed. The video showed three different conflict situations involving African American adolescents. Each scene emphasized a different aspect of conflict resolution, such as how to receive aggressive behavior, how to respond, and how to resolve conflict through negotiation and compromise. The video illustrated a conflict situation that was badly handled and then showed the same situation handled in a more effective and appropriate manner. Following the video illustrations, the group discussed the material and practiced the skills using role-playing.

A leader's manual provided detailed instructions, guidelines, and exercises for the leader. One limitation of this program turned out to be that some of the Caucasian and non–African American residents dismissed the approach as not relevant to them because the video used only adolescents of color. Currently, the anger management group uses a semi-structured approach involving role-playing and group discussion. The focus is on helping the participants identify the triggers for their anger, learning ways to delay impulsive responding, learning alternatives to physical violence, and developing assertive and other communication skills to replace maladaptive behaviors.

Topical Workshops

These are 1-day structured programs provided at different times during the year. Consultants and other experts from the outside conduct these group presentations that focus on issues such as sexual awareness, vocational issues, and other specific areas of life adjustment.

Other Groups

Other groups that have been used in the program include *parents' groups* to guide parents on how to more effectively deal with their sons on weekend passes and when they return home, and *aftercare* groups to help the residents cope with the transition from residential placement back to their homes and communities.

Sexual Offenders Treatment Program

Ocean Tides has a special Juvenile Sexual Offenders Treatment program. Residents with sexual assault charges are assigned to this program and meet in a special group. For their own protection, the specific nature of their charges is kept confidential and the residents in the program are instructed to not tell other residents the true nature of their charges, but to indicate they have nonsexual-based charges, such as assault, larceny, and so on. A consulting clinical psychologist with special expertise in working with sexual offenders conducts the sexual offenders group. Nora Sargent, PhD, has been the consultant to this program. She is a licensed clinical psychologist in full-time private practice that deals exclusively with sexual offenders. Dr. Sargent coleads the sexual offenders group with another Ocean Tides staff member, usually the director of treatment. The group is an ongoing structured group that requires a number of written assignments. These written assignments are reviewed by one of the group leaders and presented to the group, who make suggestions for changes and revisions. After the group reviews the assignment, it is rewritten and presented again to the group. This process is repeated until the group agrees that the resident has fully completed the assignment. When that acceptance is granted, the resident presents the assignment to his social worker for review and comments. The resident must continue to make adjustments to the assignment until the group leader, group, and social worker all approve it. When the assignment is finally accepted, the resident shares the finished product with his parent(s) or guardian(s) in a family session. The resident reports to the group what comments the family made. Once the assignment has received approval from the treatment group, leader, and social worker, the resident moves on to the next assignment.

The written assignments include the following:

1. *Lifeline*: A chart of the resident's life, beginning at birth and identifying all important events that have taken place in his lifetime
2. *Genogram (family tree)*: A chart identifying each member of the resident's family and anyone else that has been or is currently a significant part of his life
3. *Offense narrative*: A description of the resident's history of sexual offense behavior
4. *Support network*: An identification of six adults who know about the resident's sexual offense and who have agreed to be a resource for the resident to talk with when he needs support, help, or just some time to talk
5. *Red flags and alternatives*: Identification of as many of the specific red flag behaviors (warnings) the resident can recall, identification of the precursors ("prequels"), and realistic short-term and long-term *alternative* behaviors the resident could practice instead
6. *Decision tree*: A diagram of the choices the resident made that led to his sexual offending behavior followed by a second diagram of what the resident now understands were alternative choices that could have been made during that time

7. *Letters*: Three letters, one each to the victim(s), the resident's family, and to someone who may have abused the resident or exposed him to domestic violence
   (a) *Letter(s) to the victim(s)*: This letter should show that the resident takes full responsibility for his sexual offense and describe specifically what he did to create the opportunity for the offense. The letter should show that the resident understands some of the issues faced by the victims of sexual offenses. The letter should let the victim know that the resident understands some of the impact that his sexual offense might have had on the victim's family. Finally, the letter should demonstrate that the resident understands his treatment needs.
   (b) *Resident's letter to his family*: This letter is to show the resident's family that he takes full responsibility for his sexual offense. The letter should indicate that the resident understands some of the specific ways in which his sexual offense affected each of his family members and to indicate what he is doing to work on his personal treatment needs and goals.
   (c) *Letter to someone who may have abused the resident or exposed him to domestic violence*: This assignment involves writing a letter to the person who abused the resident (sexually, physically, and/or emotionally). The letter should tell the person what the resident now understands about the dynamics of victimization and let the person know how his or her abuse affected the resident. Also, the letter should express how the resident has been able to move on with his life and change from being a "reactor" to someone who is making healthy choices and developing healthy relationships.
8. *Relapse prevention workbook*: Satisfactorily completing all of the chapters in the workbook and sharing each chapter's exercises with appropriate members of the network
9. *Understanding my offense pattern*: The resident completes all the sections of the exercise "Understanding My Offense Pattern."
10. *Additional homework*: Completion of any other assignments given to the resident in group, by the consultant or other group leader, or by the resident's social worker

In addition to the aforementioned work in the Sexual Offenders Treatment Program, the resident is required to participate in an Anger

TABLE 5.2
Frequency of Sexual Assaults

	n	PERCENTAGE OF ALL OT BOYS	PERCENTAGE OF ALL SEXUAL ASSAULTS
Isolated incident only	63	4.0	59.4
A few times against at least one victim	33	2.1	31.1
Often against at least one victim	10	0.6	9.4

OT, Ocean Tides.

Management Group, Social Skills Training Group, Sexual Education Group, and a group that focuses on alcohol and drug education.

In terms of the boys' sexual offense charges, 4.9% ($n = 78$) of them had official sexual assault charges against them (this includes a few who incurred those charges while at Ocean Tides) and 6.7% ($n = 106$) of the boys at Ocean Tides had sexually assaulted at least one victim in his lifetime (that we are aware of). This means that the extent to which we are aware, 28 boys (1.8% of the sample) had sexually assaulted someone but were not officially charged with that offense. These boys were charged with other offenses. Considering all boys who sexually assaulted anyone whether or not he was officially charged, 12 boys (out of everyone in the whole sample) had sexually assaulted more than one victim. In terms of repeat offending, Table 5.2 illustrates that nearly 60% of all sexual assaults were isolated incidents. This table has no multiple count of boys. The most serious assault was counted for each boy, so if someone had one isolated incident and one recorded as "often," then only "often" was counted for this table.

SPECIAL PROGRAMS

Community Service

The Project SITE (Social Insight Through Experience) program provides the residents with the opportunity to provide community service by volunteering at nursing homes, day-care and preschool facilities, programs for the developmentally disabled, and comparable programs. Teachers offer individual instruction in reading, photography, music, and typing.

Project SITE is an experiential learning program in which residents earn school credit by working in the community. The underlying philosophy is that the residents can enhance their own feelings of self-esteem by helping others. Project SITE affords the residents an opportunity to provide services to the elderly, young children, and developmentally disabled people in the community through volunteer services at various agencies. Placement sites include nursery and preschools, day-care centers, nursing homes, a general hospital, and sheltered workshops for developmentally disabled adults.

Only certain residents participate in this program and they go in small groups. Agency staff provide supervision and guidance. In addition to the supervision provided by the agency, an Ocean Tides staff member acts as the group leader and accompanies them to the site. The staff member serves as a role model and helps the residents deal with any difficulties that might arise. The residents share their experiences in the group discussions following site visits. These discussions provide an opportunity for interpersonal support and problem solving. In addition, the residents keep a weekly journal that includes a description of their activities, their personal feelings about their work, and any insights they might have about the impact of their volunteer activities on themselves. As many of the youngsters in the program have impulse control problems, these discussions and the journal help to develop self-awareness and reflection. SITE participants receive positive feedback from the people they work with, agency staff, and Ocean Tides staff. The residents become aware of competencies they may not have realized that they possessed and develop feelings of accomplishment. Feelings of self-worth may become strengthened by having new labels such as "helper" and "teacher" replace old labels such as "punk," "juvenile delinquent," and "troublemaker." By working with persons that have undeveloped or diminished capacities, the young men have the opportunity to realize that they have something positive to give others. They learn that it is possible for them to succeed in school and in the community and this strengthens their self-concepts. Project SITE attempts to demonstrate to the delinquent youngster that learning can be a positive, enjoyable, and meaningful experience and is more than a boring or hated academic chore.

Field Trips

A variety of field trips also offer the opportunity for exposure to the community. Many of the residents have never traveled outside of their communities and/or neighborhoods. The highlight of the year, in terms of field trips, is an annual trip to Washington, DC, for those students who have earned it. This is a weeklong trip in which the students visit the capitol, meet with the senators and representatives from Rhode Island, and visit some of the main attractions in the nation's capital, such as Congress and the Smithsonian. At the end of each academic year, teachers offer several trips or activities that provide the students with an opportunity for a new learning experience. Examples of trips include biking, fishing, a trip to Boston, and visiting an aquarium or a museum. All trips require advance approval and include a ratio of no more than five students per teacher. All the field trips provide the residents with the opportunity to have fun, broaden their perspectives, and to participate in experiences that many of them have never had.

Summer Jobs

A particularly important skill for delinquent youngsters to learn is how to make money honestly and through legitimate employment. Ocean Tides offers a comprehensive program in which residents can work at jobs both on and off the campus. Jobs include a variety of tasks on the property, such as landscaping, maintenance, and housekeeping. Federal and other foundation grants provide the money to fund these summer positions. Ocean Tides staff members supervise the on-campus jobs. Some local businesses, such as restaurants, employ selected residents in the summer. On-site supervisors complete rating scales that evaluate job performance (e.g., punctuality, care of tools and equipment, quality of work, and industriousness); interpersonal behavior (e.g., how well the resident gets along with coworkers, willingness to help others, use of appropriate language, and good communication skills); and response to supervision (following directions, ability to admit mistakes and to accept correction, and willingness to ask for help). Income that the young men earn from their summer employment is deposited into individual bank accounts in their names. They can withdraw money as needed with approval of the staff. Most of the funds remain in their accounts and they receive it when they complete the program. Residents who are not eligible for paid employment and those who have lost their jobs work at nonpaying jobs on campus.

Wilderness Program

Although no longer currently operational, a wilderness program existed for many years. The purpose of this program was similar to Outward Bound programs with two specific goals: (a) to increase feelings of self-esteem, competence, and self-reliance by developing basic skills in hiking, mountaineering, rock climbing, backpacking, and camping; and (b) to teach the importance of interpersonal cooperation in mastering survival skills. Additional goals were to increase the youngsters' awareness of outdoor recreational activities available in the northeastern United States and to instill a respect for the natural environment. The wilderness program was composed of two related but separate activities: technical rock climbing and backpacking. Ocean Tides staff that were trained and experienced climbers provided classroom and field instruction in rock climbing. Instructions included (a) the use of equipment, such as the rope and knots, carabiners, and descenders; and (b) climbing techniques, such as anchors, the belay, signals, and the rappel. Youngsters participated in rock-climbing activities at close and accessible boulder outcroppings. In the summer, the staff led 5-day backpacking trips to the White Mountain National Forest in New Hampshire. All residents in the program were rotated through in small groups. The backpacking trips provided the opportunity for the residents to use the various outdoor skills that they learned in the classroom during the year, such as orienteering or how to travel by map and compass. Residents learned what equipment and clothing were necessary, what food to take, and how to pack a backpack. Finally, residents learned how to hike safely, disposing of waste in an environmentally protective manner (carry in–carry out), and dealing with unpredictable weather in the mountains. For the majority of the residents, these wilderness activities were a totally new experience. Many of them had never been out of an urban environment.

CONCLUSIONS

In summary, Ocean Tides provides a carefully structured program that features individualized education in an excellent school, individual and family counseling, closely supervised residential life, and a variety of recreational activities for the residents. The staff and administrators are regularly evaluated to ensure the maintenance of high standards of care. The residents are closely monitored to evaluate their progress. The program offers a variety of special activities to help the residents develop useful personal and social skills, increase their awareness of the world outside of their own environmental backgrounds, and provide them with new experiences. All of these aspects of the program are designed to reduce unnecessary strain and help raise the young men's levels of self-esteem and provide them with positive alternatives to delinquency and criminal activities. In the next chapter, the authors discuss in greater detail how the program works with the residents to bring about the necessary changes in their lives.

REFERENCES

Guerra, N. G., Kim, T. E., & Boxer, P. (2008). What works: Best practices for juvenile offenders. In R. D. Hoge, N. G. Guerra, & P. Boxer (Eds.), *Treating the juvenile offender* (pp. 79–102). New York, NY: Guilford Press.

Hammond, W. R., & Yung, B. R. (1991). *Dealing with anger: Givin' it, takin' it, workin' it out: A violence prevention program for African American youth.* Champaign, IL: Research Press.

Lehane, D. (2010). *Moonlight mile.* New York, NY: HarperCollins.

Lindner, C., & Wagner, R. (1983). The Ocean Tides experiment: Treatment of serious juvenile offenders in an open residential setting. *Federal Probation, 47*(1), 26–32.

Ocean Tides. (1988). *Social services department handbook.* Narragansett, RI: Ocean Tides.

CHAPTER 6

Calming Seas: Managing the Ocean Tides Residents

REHABILITATING YOUTHFUL OFFENDERS

Residential placement is indicated when a youngster becomes unmanageable at home, when outpatient- or community-based treatment does not work, or when it is mandated by the court. Many juveniles who have been found delinquent by a juvenile or family court judge are committed to some type of correctional facility. As Shoemaker (2009) notes, these long-term institutions have traditionally been known as *industrial schools*, *reform schools*, or *training schools*. He further points out that other kinds of facilities exist, such as *forestry camps*, *wilderness programs*, *ranches*, or other *challenge* facilities, but these are relatively rare in comparison with the total number of juvenile institutions in the United States. In addition, there are community-based correctional institutions such as *group homes* and *halfway houses*. Despite the predominance of residential-based correctional facilities, Guerra, Kim, and Boxer (2008) point out that "there are few proven treatment programs for delinquent youth and no proven program models in custodial settings" (the authors cite Greenwood, 2006, as their source for this conclusion). They indicate that two of the three types of intervention programs that have been found, on the basis of empirical research, to be effective in delinquency prevention and treatment involve family counseling. With regard to the family meetings and family counseling, it is important to note that the social services staff do not use the more formal or traditional approaches to family therapy, such as structural family therapy (Minuchin, 1974; Minuchin & Fishman, 1981); strategic family therapy

(Haley, 1972, 1976; Haley & Hoffman, 1967); or other theoretical models. Because of a whole variety of problems with these families, traditional approaches to family therapy do not work well and the goals of intervention are more modest. Instead, the social services staff uses a more eclectic and practical approach that combines aspects of different approaches (Grebstein, 1986).

Principles of Rehabilitation

In discussing the successful rehabilitation of juvenile delinquents, Romig (1978) emphasizes that the focus should be on teaching the delinquents skills "that have been documented as improving their subsequent community behavior" (Romig, 1978, p. 109). According to Romig (1978), these skills are general areas of rehabilitation that can help all delinquent youths. Romig (1978, p. 109) groups these skills into the general areas of daily living and survival skills, communication skills, the development of study skills that can lead to obtaining a diploma or certificate that will help achieve career goals, and learning career decision-making and problem-solving skills. Romig (1978, p. 109) emphasizes the importance of using effective teaching methods that include setting specific behavioral and learning goals; individualizing the presentation of information that is based on personally relevant material; teaching basic academic skills, sequential presentation of information, breaking complex skills into simple steps; using positive reinforcement by initially rewarding youngsters' attention and persistence; differential reinforcement of learning performance; and using multisensory techniques. It is important for students to have the opportunity to practice their skills outside the classroom in problem settings or actual job situations. In addition to working with the youngsters, it is essential to provide family training in communication, problem-solving, and disciplining skills.

Criteria for Effective Treatment Programs

To be considered as a treatment program of proven effectiveness, Guerra et al. (2008) list three criteria: programs that have been carefully evaluated with offenders in multiple settings and include longer term outcomes; programs that have been reviewed by a scientific advisory group; and programs that are used wisely, suggesting cost-effectiveness and feasibility. According to Guerra et al. (2008), only three programs meet these criteria: multisystem family therapy (Hengeller, Schoenwald, Borduin, Rowland, & Cunningham, 1998); functional family therapy (FFT; Alexander & Parsons, 1973); and multidimensional foster care. These authors note further that there is very limited evidence for effective intervention programs, particularly for incarcerated youngsters. Although FFT has demonstrated its efficacy with a range of delinquency-related behaviors (Sexton & Turner, 2010), almost all of the studies are community based and relatively few of them have been conducted with either incarcerated youth or delinquents with serious felony charges. Of the 27 studies cited by Alexander, Waldron, Robbins, and Neeb (2013), only five involve post-incarcerated delinquents with serious or felony charges. The remainder of the research has been with delinquents charged with status offenses, misdemeanors, habitual truancy, and substance abuse or running away.

Based on their review of the empirical evidence from multiple program evaluations, Guerra et al. (2008) cite four critical components for effective programming: (a) highly structured interventions are more effective than unstructured programs; (b) interventions that include a cognitive component that is linked to specific skills are more effective; (c) effective interventions involve families and reduce familial risk for delinquency; and (d) comprehensive interventions that address multiple risk factors across different contexts work better than single-component programs (Guerra, Kim, & Boxer, 2008, p. 87).

Essential Components for Successful Residential Treatment

The most effective residential program then should include components devoted to education, the management of daily life, personal and family counseling, special programs that build social skills, extension houses for proper transition back into the community, and aftercare. Lerner (2005, p. 31) refers to what he calls the "big three" as essential elements of optimal youth development programs. He hypothesized that these three elements are: "(1) that the contact with the adolescent is positive and sustained (for at least one year; Rhodes, 2002); (2) involves adult-youth relationships; and, (3) includes skill building activities and opportunities to use these skills by participating in, and leading, community-based activities."

Education

Delinquent youngsters often turn to antisocial behavior because of lack of competencies, skills, and knowledge in socially acceptable and conventional areas. They frequently do not like school, regardless of their intelligence or cognitive abilities, and often do not do well (46.8% of the Ocean Tides boys had performed consistently poorly throughout school). In many cases, they have fallen behind their peers by failing one or more grades and have lost motivation to learn (55.8% of the Ocean Tides boys reported consistently poor motivation for academic pursuits prior to entering the program). It is important for these youngsters to receive enough education to be eligible for employment, specific vocational training, or continued education. This requires an educational program that is sufficiently flexible to provide the individualized attention that these students may need. The school should be able to offer small classes; skilled and creative teachers; tutors, teachers' aides, or other support staff; and a curriculum that is perceived as relevant and useful by the students. The school should be able to offer remediation in basic skills such as reading and math for the less-skilled students and the opportunity to do double credits or make up work for the better-skilled students. Ideally, the school should be an accredited high school so that students are eligible to return to public school without penalty or, in the case of seniors, can continue on to higher education if they are so inclined.

Management of Daily Life

Although often possessing considerable "street smarts," juvenile delinquents are frequently lacking in the practical skills of daily living. They do not know how to cook, serve meals, behave appropriately at meal times, maintain personal hygiene, do laundry and other housekeeping tasks, participate in sports or other organized recreational activities, and interact with each other in socially appropriate ways. To learn these skills requires a competent and well-trained residential staff who can both model and supervise these activities. The staff is responsible for closely monitoring and supervising the youngsters to ensure that the residents follow the program's rules and that they interact in a socially appropriate manner. Competent helpers can fail for lack of an effective program structure. Similarly, well-designed programs can fail because of the shortcomings of individual staff members. These youngsters often have a history of interpersonal conflict with peers, arguing, fighting, bullying, scapegoating and harassment, stealing, and poor impulse control. Dealing with behaviors in a corrective and nonpunitive manner requires considerable skill, tact, and patience on the part of the residential staff.

Personal and Family Counseling

Adolescents in general are often portrayed as being in a state of constant emotional upheaval and unwilling to communicate with adults in a socially appropriate manner. Although research has shown that this stereotype is inaccurate for most adolescents and is probably only true for troubled adolescents, incarcerated juvenile delinquents generally fall into the troubled category. These youngsters often experience personal conflicts, worries and emotional problems, and have difficult family situations ranging in severity from mildly dysfunctional to inconceivable. The old adage that the apple does not fall too far from the tree holds true in that troubled children often share many characteristics with their parents that make effective parent–child communication difficult (Plomin, Chipuer, & Loehlin, 1990). Likewise, negative parenting is exacerbated by the bad behavior of adolescents. Counseling one and not the other can be ineffective.

Despite their need for counseling, these youngsters are often highly resistant to any efforts to provide help because they perceive any sort of mental health intervention as highly stigmatizing. Prior to their sentencing, many of these youngsters have been exposed to the opportunity for outpatient counseling and have either refused to participate or been noncompliant with treatment. They have significant disdain for any process that is likely to label them as emotionally disturbed or abnormal. Although they need counseling, getting them to participate in it can be a challenge. An effective program must have regular counseling available to the youngsters and their families on an ongoing basis while they are in residence. Effective counseling with these youngsters and their families requires more direct involvement by the counselor. Rather than focusing on psychological insight and introspection, the emphasis is on identifying troublesome situations and teaching practical problem-solving skills. The counselor often has to take primary responsibility for initiating and maintaining the counseling contacts, including making home visits to involve the families. Regular family counseling while the youngster is in residence is important for successful return to the community once the residential program has been completed.

Special Programs

The opportunity to be involved in enjoyable, challenging, productive, and socially sanctioned activities provides one of the main sources for positive self-esteem. Juvenile delinquents often lack the skills and/or opportunities to participate in such activities and their delinquent acts have become an alternative source of emotional gratification. An effective residential program should provide opportunities for participating in special activities to enhance the self-esteem and skill development of its residents. Examples of such positive activities include, but are not limited to, participation in competitive athletics with other schools and programs; field trips; wilderness and overnight camping programs; supervised volunteer activities to nursing and assisted-living facilities for the aged and to preschools; part-time paid jobs and summer employment; and internships, apprenticeships, and comparable opportunities for vocational training.

Extension Houses

Going from a highly structured and closely supervised residential program to the community is a difficult adjustment. This transition can be facilitated by an intermediate placement in a less-structured extension house. The extension houses are comparable to facilities that are more commonly referred to as group homes or halfway houses. Extension houses usually are private homes in the community that have been purchased and remodeled to accommodate a small number of residents (five to nine) and supervisory staff. This placement provides the opportunity for greater personal freedom and more autonomy of functioning while still requiring staff supervision. At these homes, residents can practice applying the daily living skills, such as housecleaning, cooking, and personal care that they learned in residence.

Aftercare

The final step in the rehabilitative process is a youngster's return to his family and the community. To ensure a smooth transition, a program should provide follow-up aftercare in which a representative of the program, usually a social services worker, maintains contact with the youngster and his family to help cope with any problems of readjustment that may arise.

OCEAN TIDES: A UNIQUE AND MODEL PROGRAM

If accurately described, Ocean Tides would be labeled as a "residential/ education/treatment, community based, and family oriented" program. From its inception, Ocean Tides has been dedicated to providing a coordinated, flexible, and individualized treatment program for each of its residents. A basic premise of the program is that the life of each youngster must be integrated in all its aspects. The goal of the program is to help a boy change his pattern of negative behavior so that he is going in a more positive direction in his life. Ocean Tides attempts to help young men face and correct their shortcomings by providing a blend of direction, affirmation, education, counseling, skill development, and nurturing care. The program provides the necessary ingredients to encourage the development of self-sufficiency, self-fulfillment, and self-efficacy that will facilitate a young man's successful return to his family and the community.

Treatment Philosophy

The basic philosophy of the Ocean Tides program is stated in its Mission Statement described in the Ocean Tides *Handbook for School Staff* (Ocean Tides, 1980, p. 2) as follows:

> Ocean Tides believes that every person referred to us is a unique individual worthy of our respect, and needing our care and attention. We believe that we assume responsibility for the growth and welfare of a fellow human being. We

> believe that each individual who comes to us has the capacity to learn and to achieve success in his personal and behavioral development. We further believe that this is accomplished through the everyday experiences and interactions of the individual with us as concerned human beings and through the program designed for the individual youngster.... Ocean Tides aims to help such a boy so that he can change direction, so that instead of going nowhere, he can be going somewhere.

As it turns out, Ocean Tides was ahead of its time in that the philosophy and goals of the program were based on a more positive and optimistic conceptualization of adolescent development and delinquent behavior that has more recently been referred to "positive youth development" (Lerner, 2005, p. 13). From this perspective, "the best way to prevent problem behaviors was to focus on adolescent strengths, not deficits, and to promote positive changes across the second decade of life."

Although this positive orientation is currently more in vogue, it was not the prevailing belief at the time of the founding of the Ocean Tides. Drawing from Lerner's (2005, p. 3) theoretical summary, the predominant conceptual orientation for the study of adolescent development since the early 1900s has been a "deficit model." He explains that youth are seen as "broken," in danger of becoming broken, or as "problems to be managed" (Lerner, 2005, p. 3). When youth behaved normatively, the absence of nonnormative behavior was emphasized instead of their positive behavior. For example, instead of emphasizing how well an adolescent performed academically or athletically, the youth would be described as not engaging in negative behaviors (e.g., not abusing drugs or alcohol or not participating in crime or violence).

Recognizing Individual Differences Among Delinquents

There are so many similarities in the backgrounds and behaviors of delinquents that there is a temptation to lump them together into a group, category, or stereotype. However, psychology's fundamental premise of individual differences holds for them as it does for all of us. Although it is important to recognize that each young man is a unique individual and to treat him accordingly, there are some characteristics common to many delinquents that suggest guidelines for their care. One common denominator of all the residents in the program is that they have committed crimes of sufficient magnitude to be sentenced by a court of law. In the case of juvenile delinquents in Rhode Island, it is the family court. In addition to their formal charges, many of these young men have histories of noncompliance with customary modes of socially acceptable behavior, including defiance, disobedience, and aggression. In addition to their antisocial behavior, many youngsters are lacking in sufficient social and learning skills to succeed in school or work, have little or no ambition to succeed in a socially acceptable manner, have little awareness of what is required to succeed in "the real world," and have little insight into their situation.

Beachaine, Hinshaw, and Pang (2010) have developed a useful model for understanding how biological vulnerability and environmental factors interact to produce antisocial personality development culminating in comorbid diagnoses of attention deficit hyperactivity disorder (ADHD) and early-onset conduct disorder. Their model is particularly relevant to our residents because at least 61% of the Ocean Tides boys exhibit some form of behavioral impulse control problems. In their model, Beachaine et al. (2010, p. 330) differentiate between youngsters with an early inherited biological risk of impulsivity who are exposed to a *high-risk environment* versus a *protective environment*. In both environments, the child begins with behavioral reactivity, impulsivity, and oppositional behavior. In the high-risk environment, the parent responds with coercive attempts at power assertion and control and negative reinforcement of arousal and aggression. This leads to repeated conflict escalation and negative reinforcement of emotional lability and anger. Inherited impulsivity is met with weak emotional regulation skills resulting in comorbid ADHD and opposition defiant disorder (ODD) and chronic mood dysregulation. This, in turn, leads to deviant peer group affiliations, exposure to neighborhood violence, criminality, and drug use. The final step is continuing comorbid ADHD and conduct disorder and antisocial personality development. In other words, the genetic vulnerability interacts with environmental risk to produce lifelong antisocial behavior.

Children fortunate enough to be exposed to a protective environment, on the other hand, have a different set of experiences and more favorable outcome. In the protective environment, parents avoid power struggles and provide calm, firm limit setting, and clear consequences for aggression. As a result, there is de-escalation of arousal, repeated conflict de-escalation, and positive reinforcement of prosocial behaviors. Consequently, inherited impulsivity is met with strong emotion regulation skills leading to healthy peer group affiliations and neighborhood cohesion. The impulsivity is socialized and the regulated impulsivity results in a diagnosis of ADHD only. In other words, if this model is accurate, children with similar genetic vulnerabilities can end up as delinquents or not, depending on the kind of environment and parenting to which they were exposed.

The challenge in any treatment or education program is to develop an effective program that provides consistent and fair guidelines for appropriate behavior, while at the same time, taking into consideration the unique personalities and needs of the individual youngsters. A program has to simultaneously provide support and recognition for positive behaviors and clear guidelines and related disciplinary measures for unacceptable or inappropriate behavior. In the context of Beachaine et al.'s (2010) model, a program has to take youngsters who were exposed to a high-risk environment and reexpose them to a protective environment with the hope that this can correct, reorient, or rehabilitate the existing antisocial behaviors.

Reality Therapy

Historically, the initial treatment philosophy at Ocean Tides was based on the principles of reality therapy (Glasser, 1965), an approach that had been developed in a school for delinquent girls in California. The basis of reality therapy is to help persons fulfill two basic needs: "the need to love and be loved and the need to feel that we are worthwhile to ourselves and to others" (Glasser, 1965, p. 9). The two key concepts in reality therapy are *relationship* and *responsibility*. Glasser (1965, p. 13) defines responsibility as: "the ability to fulfill one's needs, and to do so *in a way that does not deprive others of the ability to fulfill their needs*." In reality therapy, responsibility is taught and developed through relationships. As Glasser (1965, p. 7) notes: "we must be involved with other people, one at the very minimum, but hopefully many more than one. At all times in our lives we must have at least one person who cares about us and whom we care for ourselves. If we do not have this essential person, we will not be able to fulfill our basic needs." According to Agnew (2005), lacking or losing this positive component will increase the likelihood that a juvenile will seek criminal opportunities to relieve the strain presented by its absence.

Relationships provide the context for change at Ocean Tides. The program is based on the belief, consistent with reality therapy, that caring by the staff is essential for successful treatment and rehabilitation. Beyond that, strong relationships serve as stakes in conformity in attempts to maintain those relationships. If the staff, both individually and collectively, can consistently communicate their caring to the resident, then a relationship(s) may begin to form that stimulates a process of change and growth in the delinquent. It takes more than words to communicate caring. Caring is conveyed through the actions and everyday behavior of the staff. Caring is demonstrated by maintaining an effective relationship, in which staff members are willing to risk unpopularity with the residents by setting limits, providing clear expectations of appropriate behavior, and providing discipline in a nonpunitive manner. In the various interpersonal interactions that occur, the young man must have a sense that he is cared for, respected, and loved. He must also come to believe that he is accountable for his decisions, that he is responsible.

Building Relationships

This is precisely what the Ocean Tides program attempts to do. The establishment of caring and trusting relationships between staff and residents is the key to successful treatment. The Ocean Tides program philosophy, as stated in the *Social Services Department Handbook* (Ocean Tides, 1988, p. 4), is as follows:

> Ocean Tides believes that every person referred to us is a unique individual worthy of our respect, and needing our care and attention. We believe that we assume responsibility for the growth and welfare of a fellow human being. We believe that each individual who comes to us has the capacity to learn and to achieve success in his/her personal and behavioral development. We further believe that this is accomplished both through the everyday experiences and interactions of the individual with us as concerned human beings and through the program developed for the individual.

Building good relationships with the residents involves several key elements on the part of the staff member. These include respect; clear and direct communication; a caring approach and positive regard for the adolescent; and fair, consistent, and appropriate limit setting. Effective supervision means adopting the role of an effective adult and role model, not a friend, pal, or buddy. Many of the residents have been exposed to ineffective parenting. They may have experienced the significant adults in their lives as behaving more like adolescents than responsible adults. Part of being a responsible and effective adult is to be able to have clear expectations for acceptable behavior, set limits, and provide fair and reasonable discipline. The core of treatment at Ocean Tides consists of having all staff—teachers, residential counselors, and social workers—act as mature adults who can provide consistent and caring treatment. They must be willing to invest the time and effort necessary to establish relationships with the residents and follow issues through. Supervision, limit setting, and discipline are informed by a caring approach and positive regard for the adolescent. Although it is important to establish relationships with the adolescents, staff members should never compromise the adult role in order to develop a relationship. Maintaining objectivity, fairness, and consistency is an important element of effective supervision and treatment.

LaSallian Heritage

Although Ocean Tides is a secular and nondenominational program, it draws heavily from the philosophy of John Baptist de La Salle, the French priest who founded the Brothers of the Christian Schools. At the time of his death in 1719, he left an institute dedicated to running schools for the poor. The mission of the LaSallian educator is the human and Christian education of youth, especially poor youth. LaSallian educators are attentive to each of their students and especially to those most in need. They make themselves available to all with the attitude of brotherly companionship. "To touch the hearts of your students . . . is the greatest miracle you can perform and the one that God asks of you, for this the purpose of your work" (Loes & Huether, 1994, p. 257, 139.3).

Treatment is considered to be an educational experience. It is analogous to what a person undergoes in physical therapy when recovering from an injury. The physical therapist provides exercises and treatments designed to strengthen and repair the damaged part of the body. The process may be painful, stressful, frustrating, and difficult. The therapist provides the guidance, instruction, encouragement, and support, but ultimately it is the patient's responsibility to do the work necessary to recover. It requires making an effort, accepting encouragement and the challenge, and tolerating the pain during the initial phase of strengthening the weakened areas. Successful therapy and recovery are based on the patient's learning to trust the therapist and himself.

Treatment at Ocean Tides is grounded in the belief that successful rehabilitation results from a combination of a good program and talented, committed people. This is achieved through the development of individual treatment plans constructed by an interdepartmental treatment team. The program is based on the assumption that a resident must learn new and more effective skills in problem solving and in self-control in order to stay out of future trouble. There is an additional assumption that a young man must improve his self-image and must learn to think better of himself and his future possibilities. His self-concept will improve and his self-esteem will increase only if he makes real achievements that are evident to him. A youngster used to criticism, failure, and "put-downs" by others requires clear external affirmation of his progress in order to alter his self-perception. In this respect, frequent and tangible feedback in the form of point sheets in class or daily written progress records about his behavior plays an important role. Equally important are the informal words of affirmation from staff. When a staff member takes the time to explain to a resident what he did wrong, it allows negative behaviors to be viewed as alterable mistakes rather than irreversible signs of a defective character or flawed personality. "I'm no good" is replaced by "I did something wrong" or "I made a mistake." As modern behavioral psychology has demonstrated, positive reinforcement through noticing and commenting on acceptable behaviors can be very effective. The other advantage of recognizing positive behavior is that it counters the tendency to use negative behavior as an attention-getting device, a practice common to delinquents.

Finally, honesty is both a goal of the program and a key to its success. When a young man begins the program, he is told that honesty with oneself and others is a key ingredient of the success of the program. The hope and belief are that honesty with oneself will lead to more effective problem solving and better control over one's life. If a young man can develop more control over the direction of his life and make better choices, the program will have been successful.

Physical Description and Location

The residential program is located on the spacious grounds of a former novitiate training center for the Christian Brothers in Narragansett, Rhode Island, a small seaside community. The campus is walking distance to popular ocean beaches. Residents have their own individual dormitory rooms that they can decorate as they wish. The grounds are spacious with ample room for outdoor sports and recreation. From the standpoint of physical comfort and attractiveness, the facility is vastly different from and a pleasant alternative to the stark institutional nature of most training schools or youth prisons. On the contrary, the facilities resemble those of a private preparatory school much more than they do a state institution. Attractive stone walls surround the property, not fences with barbed or razor wire on top.

Until recently, there were "extension" houses in addition to the main residential campus. These were community-based group homes. Originally, there were four such group homes, but all of them gradually had to be closed because of state budget cuts. Three of the houses were located in the greater metropolitan area of the capital city. The fourth house was in a smaller community halfway between the main residential campus and the capital city. These houses served as intermediary placements for the youngsters before they returned to the community. The extension house provides a smaller and less-structured environment that serves as an intermediary adjustment period to returning home. Youngsters in placement at the group home are responsible for daily living skills, such as cooking and cleaning, under the supervision of residential staff. An alternative to being placed in an extension house and a fourth option for residents is to live in the "honor dormitory." This is a separate residential area comprising only six rooms that is located in a separate dormitory area on the grounds of the main residential campus.

The main residential campus is divided into two main areas: the school and the residential area. The school is a modern, well-equipped facility consisting of classrooms, a library, a computer room, art room and kiln for ceramics, a science laboratory, a woodshop, and an adjacent room for wood-turning classes. In addition to the school facilities, there is a large conference room and a smaller conference room and individual offices for the principal and social services staff. The residential area consists of dormitory rooms, TV lounge, and gymnasium with adjacent weight training room, including a heavy punching bag, and a pool table. The dormitory rooms are located on hallways that can be locked so that residents do not have access to the dormitory rooms during the school day.

Referrals to Ocean Tides

All referrals to the program originate with the state Department of Children, Youth and Families (DCYF) Residential Review Team. In order to be eligible for the program, a young man must be court adjudicated and have been found guilty of legal offenses. Residents come either from the state training school or have been ordered into placement by the family court. The family court makes some referrals to Ocean Tides directly or as a condition of probation. Residents who have been referred from the training school were in a regular residential unit or in a temporary detention unit for youth awaiting placement in another facility. Youngsters coming from the training school are on Temporary Community Placement (TCP) at Ocean Tides from the training school. Social workers or other responsible personnel at the training school refer youngsters who they think could benefit from placement at Ocean Tides.

Intake Process

Once a referral is received, the Administrative Intake Committee reviews all the written information on each youngster. They advise the president–director of treatment as to the appropriateness of the referral. The next step is to interview the youngster. If the young man is a resident at the training school, he is interviewed there. Youngsters referred as a condition of probation come to Narragansett with their probation counselor for an interview. The Intake Committee makes a decision based on the written referral material and the interview and advises the president–director of treatment, who is responsible for making the final decision for admission to the program or rejection.

Daily Routines

The Ocean Tides program is designed to provide a safe and secure environment where the adolescents feel comfortable enough to try out new behaviors and make changes in their lives. The program attempts to accomplish this through a structured approach with clear schedules, routines, activities, rules, and limits on unacceptable behavior.

The day begins at 7:25 a.m. when a staff member wakes up each youngster. Residents have individual bedrooms located adjacent to each other in a dormitory section.

The residents have until 8:15 a.m. to shower and place their breakfast orders to prepare for breakfast. Before leaving the dorm, each resident must shower, make his bed, pick up any trash or clothing from the floor, lock his closet and secure all valuables, turn off the light, and close his door. Residents must eat all the hot food that they order from the grill or they will not be allowed to order hot food the following day. This is referred to as being "Off Grill" or OG. Residents may always eat cereal, toast, and juice. Residents take turns acting as servers for meals. The breakfast servers report to the kitchen at 8:00 a.m. and the rest of the residents go up to the dining room at 8:25 a.m. After breakfast, residents return to the dormitory area to brush their teeth, change into their school uniforms, and get anything they need from their rooms. Residents remain in their rooms until they are called for school, which begins at 9:30 a.m.

All residents attend school from 9:30 a.m. to 3:30 p.m. After school, the residential staff have a brief meeting with all of the residents to inform them of the schedule for the remainder of the afternoon and evening. After the meeting, recreation begins and continues until 4:45 p.m. The purpose of recreation is to get some exercise, fresh air, learn teamwork, have some fun, and to help provide a break between school and the evening activities. Participation in recreation is mandatory unless a resident is ill. Some examples of recreational activities include flag football, softball, soccer, basketball, scatter ball, hockey, weight lifting, swimming at the beach in the summer, walks, and trips to playgrounds (i.e., outdoor basketball courts). After recreation ends, residents have a brief time in the dormitory when they can take a quick shower with staff permission. From the end of recreation until dinner is generally a free time for residents in which they can do schoolwork, use the gym, watch

TV, play cards, do sanctions, and so on. If a resident has sanction time, he may not participate in privilege activities, such as pool, ping-pong, video games, DVD movies, and so on, until he completes the sanctions. During the school year, residents are usually required to watch at least a portion of the local evening news. They may have math or reading tutoring at some point in the evening.

Dinner is served at 6:15 p.m. After dinner, there is free time until a brief evening meeting followed by snacks. Different activities are planned for each evening of the week. These activities include DVD movies, trips to the local university swimming pool, organized basketball games, educational groups (e.g., substance abuse and sexuality), movie trips, and cookouts in the summer. After evening activities are concluded, residents return to their dorm rooms to prepare for bed. Lights must be shut off at 10:30 p.m. and radios turned off no later than 11 p.m.

Weekends

Weekends are slightly less structured and more relaxed due to the smaller number of residents and more free time. However, all of the usual responsibilities and expectations for good behavior remain the same. There are two different categories of weekend residents. The first is those new residents who are still on orientation. The second is residents who have lost the weekend pass for disciplinary reasons. This latter group participates in a work program that consists of doing housework and other chores on the property as determined by the staff. Residents participating in the work program are usually not allowed off grounds for the Saturday night movie or for their Sunday family visit.

Home Passes

After successfully completing the orientation period of 5 weeks, residents can *earn* weekend home visits. Home passes are a privilege and depend on the residents' cooperation with the total program. Attitude and behavior during previous home passes are also taken into consideration. Each resident's social services counselor contacts the parents or other approved adult pass resource each Thursday to provide them with information about the weekend pass. If the social services counselor is not able to contact the parents on Thursday, the young man will not be sent home until direct parent contact has occurred.

Home passes usually begin on Friday afternoons after school ends. Ocean Tides has vans that transport the boys from the Narragansett Campus to a designated spot in downtown Providence (the capital city). During the school year, the arrival time is usually between 4:30 p.m. and 5:00 p.m. Arrival time may differ in the summer and on special days (e.g., end of a school quarter and distribution of report cards day). The resident and his parents should arrange transportation from the drop-off spot in Providence to the home. Return to Ocean Tides occurs on Sunday night when the van picks up the boys at a designated location at 8:30 p.m. At certain times during the year, such as public holidays and school vacations, residents may be permitted to have extended home visits.

If a resident misses the van on the return trip, he or his parents are instructed to call the Narragansett Campus immediately and inform them. It then becomes the parents' responsibility to arrange transportation. Under no circumstances is the resident allowed to remain at home. If the young man is on TCP from the training school and is more than 2 hours late in returning from a weekend pass, the authorities will be notified that he is AWOL from the program. Returning late from a weekend pass will also affect the length of his next weekend pass. If a resident has any involvement with the police during a home visit, Ocean Tides should be notified immediately. If a police department files formal charges against a resident, his home visits will be suspended until these charges have been resolved.

Weekend Rules

An important part of the home visit is to allow the resident time to spend with his family and in his community so that the relationship between the resident and his family can be strengthened. The social services counselor will help the parents to establish a curfew for each night that the resident is home. If there is a small violation of this curfew, parents should make some adjustment in the curfew for the following evening. Similarly, if there are minor behavioral problems on the weekend, parents are expected to take suitable disciplinary action. The program does not want to diminish or interfere with the parents' authority. However, if the curfew and rules are not respected on a consistent basis, Ocean

Tides will become involved. This behavior could result in loss of part or the entire next weekend pass. Ocean Tides sets a curfew of 11:00 p.m. for those residents in the program as a condition of probation. All residents on TCP from the Rhode Island Training School have a curfew of 11:00 p.m. set by the Juvenile Parole Unit. Ocean Tides enforces curfews by random curfew calls made each weekend by the administrator on call. When a resident receives a curfew call, he must be available to speak directly to the administrator. A missed curfew call occurs when the resident is not at home, if the phone is busy, if there is no answer, or if a machine answers. If the administrator does not speak directly to the resident for any reason, the resident will lose part of the next weekend pass. There are no exceptions to this rule. Repeated missed curfew calls will result in more serious consequences. During weekend passes, residents must sleep at home. No exceptions can be made without prior approval from Ocean Tides through the social services counselor. The penalty for violating this rule is partial loss of the next weekend pass. Finally, residents are not allowed to spend time together during weekend passes. Violation of this rule will result in losing part or the entire next weekend pass.

Weekend Sheet

In order to obtain information about the resident's progress during a weekend pass, it is important that the parent or responsible caretaker take time to complete the weekend sheet with honest comments about both the positive and negative points of the visit. These forms are very important in evaluating a resident's progress in the program. It is the resident's responsibility to return this form. Failure to return the weekend sheet results in the following consequences: (a) the first time the form is not returned, the resident receives a warning from his social services counselor; (b) the second time the form is not returned, the resident receives a late van and does not leave Ocean Tides until 9:00 a.m. on Saturday; (c) the third time, the resident's departure is delayed until Saturday afternoon; and (d) on the fourth and all future occasions, failure to return the weekend sheet results in loss of the weekend home visit. If the parents misplace the weekend sheet, they can write a note describing how the weekend went. If they forget or refuse to complete the sheet, the boys return the empty form.

Structuring Cooperative Behavior

In an attempt to rehabilitate the residents and teach them appropriate social skills, there are a number of specific guidelines that are detailed in the various departmental handbooks that residents receive. In general, these guidelines describe what is considered normal and appropriate behavior in social situations. For example, there is no smoking, betting, gambling, or trading allowed. Residents must shower each morning and dress appropriately. Shoes and shirts must be worn at all times in the dining room. Residents are expected to be polite to servers and to display proper dining room etiquette. There is no cursing or vulgar talk, and personal items, such as an iPod and other listening devices, are not allowed in the dining room. When residents are on off-campus excursions, they must remain within staff sight and exhibit mature and appropriate behavior. When on a beach walk, residents are not allowed to make contact with any person who is not associated with Ocean Tides. Horseplay and fooling around by residents are prohibited when being transported in a van or when on a field trip or other excursion.

Social Skills and Peer Issues

Delinquent young men typically have difficulty in their peer relationships. One of the reasons delinquents tend to hang out together is that nondelinquent peers often avoid them and do not want to have anything to do with them. Delinquents have trouble relating to others and each other because they lack the rudimentary social skills necessary for successful interpersonal interaction. Poor frustration tolerance, lack of empathy, and lack of verbal skills are often replaced by verbally and physically aggressive behavior. In view of this, how well do the residents at Ocean Tides get along with each other? Of the 1,585 young men included in the study, we have information for 1,462 (92.2%) of them. A total of 40.5% (n = 592) "gets along very well all or most of the time"; 40.1% (n = 601) "gets along well with some and not so well with others"; 1.8% (n = 27) "gets along well with peers, but has trouble with one"; 14.7% (n = 215) "does not get along with most" (of their peers); and 1.8% (n = 27) "does not get along with any" (of their peers).

The residents enter the Ocean Tides program with several interpersonal difficulties, some of which are listed in Table 2.3 in Chapter 2.

In residence, common conflicts include boys fighting over a seat or a TV show and disagreements with staff members. Although actual fights are rare, posturing and challenging behavior are not. Each conflict situation requires a calm and reasonable adult response. The residents depend on the staff to act as mature adults, to take charge, and to control the situation. Suggestions in the *Group Living Staff Handbook* (Ocean Tides, 2011) for handling difficult situations include:

1. Knowing what you expect and communicating this clearly, calmly, and firmly
2. Avoiding communicating doubt and indecision
3. Giving consequences for failure to meet your expectations

Often, prevention is the key to success. Anticipating an approaching conflict is the best way to prevent a situation from escalating. Early intervention will usually prevent a full-scale blowup from occurring. It is usually effective to separate the combatants and ask each resident separately for their perceptions of what is going on and how they are feeling.

Confronting a resident with regard to inappropriate behavior is both an extremely important skill and an inescapable responsibility for a staff member. The first step in the process is for the staff member to make his or her expectations clear at the outset. Common infractions include inappropriate language in the dining room, putting shoes on furniture, and not wanting to participate in some mandatory program activity, such as housework or recreation. Although all residents are given a handbook that clearly outlines expectations and required behavior on entering the program, noncompliance is common. It is essential that residents be made aware of inappropriate or unacceptable behavior when it occurs. Whenever possible, the adolescent is confronted at the lowest level possible (i.e., when minor infraction occur, such as putting shoes on furniture) in a manner that is nonthreatening by using calm, clear, and direct communication. The goal is to correct the behavior in a way that minimizes the likelihood of escalation into a major power confrontation between the resident and the staff member.

Low-level confrontation sends an important message to the adolescent, namely, that the staff member is not afraid to require the resident to follow the rules and that he or she cares enough to address the situation before it becomes more serious. The staff member must be careful to respond to the behavior rather than to the emotion it elicits. It goes without saying that this requires patience and a high level of frustration tolerance on the part of the staff member. It is essential that the staff member avoid the trap of allowing the resident to escalate a minor situation into a major power confrontation.

Conflicts are not only inevitable, but some may be desirable for therapeutic purposes. For example, a young man who is displacing anger from home by taking it out on a smaller or younger resident may be encouraged to express his feelings to staff members. This allows the emotions to be dealt with in a more constructive manner. In other instances, angry and sad youngsters will occasionally break things, such as furniture or doors. These youngsters might be encouraged to yell, scream, hit a pillow, or go to the gym and hit the heavy bag. Our adolescents have trouble expressing their feelings and they often hold them in until the "breaking point." This leads to considerable stress. There are a number of positive physical outlets available to the residents, such as playing basketball, ping-pong, weight lifting, and hitting the heavy bag. Residents are encouraged to use these activities to alleviate stress.

Management of Assaultive Behavior

On those rare occasions when it is necessary to intervene with an assaultive youngster or to break up an actual physical fight, the intervention is based on the following guidelines:

1. To prevent the youngster from harming himself
2. To prevent the youngster from harming others

All interventions are done in such a way as to protect the youngster and the staff member from physical harm. Although these situations are emotionally and physically taxing, in any instance where a resident loses control, a staff member's primary responsibility is to protect the adolescent. Although residential staff members have been trained in the use of restraints, restraints are not used at Ocean Tides except as a last resort in a situation in which a restraint is the only way to protect a youngster from harming himself or someone else.

Drug Screen Policy

Some residents, especially those with a documented history of drug use, may be required by order of the family court to participate in substance abuse counseling. As part of that counseling, urine screens may be required. The urine screens are conducted by an outside agency specializing in substance abuse treatment. There are consequences for "dirty" or positive urine screens. The results of the initial urine screen are used as a baseline level. The resident does not lose weekend time if the initial screen is positive. If the resident's level in subsequent screens continues to decrease at a reasonable rate (the counselor will make a determination of what is reasonable), the adolescent does not lose weekend time. If, however, levels in subsequent screens remain the same, increase, or decrease more slowly than what is reasonable, the resident loses weekend time following the receipt of the screen results. If the initial screen is positive, decreases at a reasonable rate to the point where the resident receives a clean or negative screen, and then the resident receives another positive screen, he loses the weekend pass following receipt of the screen results. A diluted drug screen is always considered to be positive and results in the loss of a weekend pass. Refusal to take a drug screen also results in the automatic loss of a weekend pass.

Searches

Although the foundation of the program's philosophy is that the individual is responsible for his own behavior, under certain circumstances, it may be necessary to search a resident. Although searching the residents and his belongings may appear to run counter to the idea of promoting individual responsibility that is the foundation of the program's philosophy, the reality is that these searches are necessary to ensure the safety of the young men and to provide a secure environment in which trust and honesty can develop. These youngsters are in residential placement because of serious prior criminal activity. In the past, they have lied, stolen, taken and sold drugs, assaulted other people, and engaged in other antisocial behavior. They cannot initially be trusted to refrain from engaging in this behavior just because they are in a residential rehabilitation program. Searches are the most practical way of preventing drugs and other potentially harmful contraband from being brought into the program.

The purpose of the searches is to avoid creating an environment in which youngsters who are genuinely interested in changing their behavior are subject to temptations that might divert them from their goals. The reality is that searches are needed for several reasons: (a) to prevent drugs, weapons, and other contraband from being brought into the program when residents return from weekend passes; (b) to prevent theft among the residents; (c) to ensure the safety of the residents; and (d) to provide a secure atmosphere in which trust and honesty can develop. A staff member may search a resident's possessions and/or a resident's room at any time deemed necessary. Many residents like to challenge authority in general and the authority of the staff in particular by "getting over" on them (i.e., having something they should not have). Searches are a practical way for staff to stay on top of those residents who wish to "get over" and to provide a positive atmosphere for those residents who are genuinely motivated to succeed in the program.

Searches are conducted individually, in privacy, and in a respectful manner as follows. When a resident returns to the campus, he must have a towel ready and be prepared to go to the shower before he is allowed to go to his room. For the search, he strips down to his underwear. Staff members use the following guidelines and procedures in conducting a search.

1. Staff members do not search a resident's body.
2. Staff members should be sensitive to the fact that strip searches are embarrassing for residents and the search should be conducted in privacy where the possibility of interruption is limited.
3. Search all articles of clothing, including trouser pockets, socks, the insides of footwear, belt buckles, underneath hat brims, trouser cuffs, shirt pockets, underwear, and so on.
4. The staff member does not have to provide a lengthy explanation regarding the reasons for conducting a search. Searches are a simple fact of life when working with juvenile offenders in a residential program.
5. Female staff members are not to conduct strip searches.
6. Be aware that the residents may be creating a suspicious situation (e.g., whispering to each other) to see if the staff member will take any action. When in doubt, conduct a search.

Disciplinary Procedures and Sanctions

An important aspect of dealing with delinquents is how to handle discipline in an effective manner. Discipline at Ocean Tides is handled through a process of sanctioning inappropriate behaviors. Although the emphasis is on acknowledging and rewarding good behavior, it is also necessary to identify and sanction unacceptable behavior. Assigning sanctions is the major method of responding to persistent unacceptable behavior by the residents when they do not respond to rational discussion of their wrongdoing. Sanctions are used only after residents have been cautioned or warned. A sanction is used as a last resort and is always preceded by a warning that if the resident does not alter his behavior, he will be sanctioned.

In the residential department, sanctions generally consist of removal from an activity, time spent alone, assignment of housework chores, or some other task that is appropriate to the offense, such as a writing assignment. Generally, the guidelines used in sanctioning behavior include (a) keeping the sanction closely related to the unacceptable behavior in time and in content, and (b) adjusting the severity of the sanction to the number of times the unacceptable behavior has occurred. Some examples are if a resident throws food in the dining room, he is assigned to clean up the dining room for a period of time; argumentative behavior, annoying others, or other disruptive behavior results in removal from the activity or location; and refusing to participate in a recreational activity can result in being assigned extra exercise.

Teachers, residential counselors, and social services counselors can administer sanctions, although the latter staff uses them less frequently. Although disciplining the adolescents through the use of sanctions is often unpleasant and stressful, sanctions are the primary tool used by staff in attempting to halt negative behaviors and replace them with more adaptive ways of interacting. Sanctions are effective when they are clear, consistent, appropriate, and "the punishment fits the crime." Following are the approved steps in sanctioning:

1. Verbal reminders
2. Remove the youngster from his peers and allow "cooling off" time
3. Verbal sanction (e.g., a simple apology)

4. Short written sanctions (e.g., a specific number of sentences or a paragraph related to the offense or assignments such as housework or other chores to be completed within a designated time period)
5. Restriction to a given area for short periods of time
6. Additional chores (extended period)
7. Loss of off-property privileges
8. Partial loss of weekend pass
9. Total loss of weekend pass(es)
10. Return to the state training school and/or family court

Sanctioning is based on the program's treatment guidelines and the discretion of the individual staff member. Examples of behaviors that are unacceptable at Ocean Tides are as follows:

- Smoking on the premises or in one's bedroom
- Not participating during recreation
- Threatening another resident
- Threatening staff
- Continued disrespect
- Being in another resident's bedroom, spitting on the floor, and so on
- Poor housework
- "Hands on" (touching another resident or staff member)
- Being out of staff sight
- Lying to staff
- "Playing" or manipulating staff
- Being anywhere without permission
- Light on in bedroom after lights out
- Late to room
- Late from the dormitory
- Fooling around or horseplay
- Unkempt or messy room, including unmade bed
- Refusing a staff request
- Shouting, yelling, or causing a disturbance in any way
- Inappropriate behavior in the dining room, kitchen, or a vehicle
- Cursing, inappropriate remarks or gestures, or talking back disrespectfully
- Feet on furniture, slamming doors, or other mistreatment of property/facilities

- Inappropriate behavior while engaging in recreational activities
- Wasting food, taking two desserts, or similar violations of proper dining behavior
- Fights, AWOL, or comparable extreme behavior

Sanction Guidelines

Staff members use the following general guidelines in assigning sanctions.

1. *Avoid audiences*: Remove the resident from his peers and deal with him individually and in private, if possible. There are many ways to do this. Consult with veteran staff about types of techniques for accomplishing this.
2. *Be aware of how you feel*: If you are tired, stressed, or upset about something else, be careful not to displace your own issues on to the resident you are sanctioning. A useful rule of thumb is not to sanction out of anger.
3. *Take time to think/discuss*: If you are upset, allow yourself and the situation to calm down before deciding on a sanction. There is no obligation to respond immediately, particularly if a hasty decision results in an unfair or overly harsh sanction. Take the time to gather your thoughts and discuss the situation with fellow staff members. Was the behavior in question really delinquent or simply immature? Remain as objective as possible. Often the delay affords the resident time to think about the situation.
4. *Avoid general reactions*: A group should not be held responsible for the actions of an individual and vice versa.
5. *Start small*: Begin with the smallest possible sanction that will be meaningful. This gives you room to move in the event the resident chooses to escalate the situation. It also allows you to hold the more serious sanctions in reserve in the event of more or continued misbehavior.
6. *Let the punishment fit the crime*: If the misbehavior took place in the TV room, revoke TV privileges; if the misbehavior occurs at the beach, remove beach privileges; if it is inappropriate dining room behavior, assign dining room cleanup tasks, and so on.

7. *Consistency and communication*: It is particularly important that all sanctions given be consistent with those given by fellow staff. Communicate with each other. Inconsistency in sanctioning by staff results in both legitimate feelings of unfairness by residents and affords them the opportunity to try and manipulate staff.
8. *Be specific*: Make every effort to be sure the resident understands exactly why he is being sanctioned. One useful technique is to ask the resident to repeat back in his own words what he did wrong. It is equally important to specifically indicate what you expect in the future. For example, "remember when you did 'A' earlier today? Maybe next time you could try 'B' if it happens again."
9. *Think treatment, not punishment*: The goal of a sanction is to change unacceptable behavior and not to express anger or frustration generated by that behavior. Vindictive behavior on the part of staff is unprofessional and inappropriate.
10. *One on one*: As noted earlier, it would be ideal if a youngster could be sanctioned separately from his peers each time he misbehaved. However, this cannot always be accomplished. Try not to reprimand a resident in front of a group. Our residents are particularly sensitive to public loss of face or being "dissed" (disrespected). A resident's perception or belief that he is being disrespected is almost certain to ignite confrontation. Indicate at the time of the infraction that the behavior is inappropriate and merits a sanction. Wait for an opportune time to correct the behavior specifically, tactfully, and firmly. Then drop it.

Residents are reminded before they leave the campus that all sanctions would be doubled for infractions that occur off-grounds.

Written Incident Reports

Whenever a situation occurs with a resident that is out of the ordinary (i.e., damages agency property, injures or attempts to injure himself or others), a formal written report is submitted to the department director who, in turn, submits it to the treatment team. The format for an incident report includes the following information: the staff member reporting; the date and time of the incident; who (names of residents) was involved; the location; a brief description of what took place and what triggered the incident; a description of the follow-up, including any sanctions given and any relevant personal observations by the staff member; and, finally, recommended sanctions. Following are a few examples of typical incident reports. To save space, the usual format has been eliminated and only the content of the reports is included.

Example 1

The following incident occurred in the TV room/hallway. "Youth received 15 minutes for poor attitude toward the present activity (movie). Youth began to have an outburst of poor language, poor staff interactions, and leaving staff sight. Youth at this time began to punch and push chairs into the walls in an outrage. Youth did calm down minutes later and was able to complete some time." *Sanctions recommended*: 3 hours and 45 minutes with additional recommended sanctions of loss of weekend time.

Example 2

"As staff members Pam and Jim were watching residents in the gym, James and Greg got into a verbal scuffle on the gym stage. Greg accidentally stepped on a ping-pong ball and James snapped at Greg for doing so. Heated words were exchanged and James escalated the fight by egging Greg to punch him. James uncontrollably stormed onto the stage, dropped multiple f-bombs, totally disrespecting staff while egging on Greg. Greg is not totally innocent; slightly instigating James." Follow-up: "James has serious anger issues. He needs to find an outlet for his anger before a serious incident occurs." *Sanctions recommended*: James: 1 hour for stepping up; 1 hour for being out of staff sight; 2 hours for severe disrespect to staff; and 0.5 hour for f-bombs.

Example 3

"After returning from dinner, we all went into the TV room. Jeff was playing cards and Andy was watching TV. Andy became very frustrated with Jeff, stating: 'This kid better stop staring at me or I'm going to bang him.' Jeff was playing cards, and from what I saw, did nothing wrong. Andy, who has a very short fuse, rushed at Jeff and was about to start a fight with him. Staff Roger got between them. Andy rushed around the couches toward the other side of Jeff and I stopped Andy from moving closer. Roger took Andy outside the TV room and the fight was over. Andy continued his out of control raging, screaming f-bombs and threats. Roger was able to calm him down and Andy went into the gym." Follow-up: "Andy has severe anger issues. I feel he needs to discuss this problem with a professional and try to get to the cause of his anger. In this instance, Jeff was not at fault. Andy received prior sanctions and was angry about them." *Sanctions recommended*: 2 hours for stepping up; 1 hour for disrespect to staff; and weekend time.

Categories of Offenses and Suggested Sanctions

Written incident reports are loosely grouped into the following categories of offenses (listed here preceded by the number and percent of boys who have received at least one sanction for each offense).

- Fighting (n = 750, 47.3%)
- Vandalism (n = 222, 14%)
- Disobedience (n = 888, 56%)
- Truancy or leaving grounds (n = 404, 25.5%)
- Disruptive to others (n = 577, 36.5%)
- Smoking pot (n = 352, 22.2%)
- Drinking alcohol (n = 160, 10%).

Suggested sanctions written into the incident reports can be categorized into the following general sanctions (listed here preceded by the number and percent of boys who have received at least one of these official sanctions).

- Housework (n = 323, 20.4%)
- Poor choice projects (n = 94, 5.9%)
- Reduced or removed time away from Ocean Tides (n = 1,159, 73.1%)
- Writing projects (n = 157, 9.9%)
- Restitution (n = 48, 3%).

New Resident Orientation

New residents undergo a 5-week orientation period. During this time, they are not allowed to go home on weekends but can have family visits. Visitors include immediate family members only. Brothers and sisters may visit but must be accompanied by a parent. All visitors are asked to sign in on arrival. No friends or girlfriends are allowed to visit. Visiting times are on Sundays from 1:00 p.m. to 5:00 p.m. During the first weekend of orientation, the visit takes place on the Ocean Tides property from 1:00 p.m. to 3:00 p.m. On the second and following weekends of orientation, parents may take residents off the property but are not allowed to go home or to their home neighborhood for any reason. Residents must remain with their parents during off-property visits.

Orientation to the program begins the moment the first staff member interacts with the resident, often starting with the trip to Ocean Tides, if the youngster is being transported from the training school. The purpose of the orientation is to familiarize the young man with the rules and procedures and to make him feel welcome. If the resident is coming directly from home, the orientation begins as soon as he arrives. The orientation consists of formal and informal procedures. Informally, staff members try to make the young man feel at ease and begin conversation with gentle inquiries about his recent experiences at home or in the training school, his interests, his expectations, and personal goals. Staff members explain some basic aspects of the program, particularly the importance of personal responsibility and honesty. After this brief introduction, a staff member takes the youngster to his room and then he takes a shower. Following his shower, the young man makes his bed and receives instructions about decorating his room.

During the orientation process, the residents meet with individual staff members from each department to discuss how each component of the program works. The young man has his own social services counselor who works with him for the duration of his stay. All initial educational and psychological testing are completed during the orientation period. In school, a standardized test of academic achievement is administered to establish a baseline. The social services worker administers a standardized personality inventory or screening test. Certain youngsters may be scheduled to meet with the consulting psychologist for an interview and brief evaluation. In addition, each youngster completes a New Student Inventory that consists of a series of simple questionnaires regarding prior school experiences, perceived educational needs and interests, and responsibility for learning. Each youngster is given a copy of the Resident's Handbook that summarizes the rules, regulations, procedures, daily activities, and expectations at Ocean Tides. A staff member explains and reviews the daily operation of the program from wake-up to bedtime. During the first weekend in residence, the youngster is encouraged to mingle with and get acquainted with the other residents. Residential staff members try to be especially attentive and sensitive to the new resident's adjustment. For example, they might talk to him about being "the new kid on the block," visit him briefly at bedtime and during quiet time, and suggest activities. Their goal is to provide reassurance and encouragement. When a new resident has trouble adjusting to the program or is uncooperative, the orientation period may be extended beyond the customary 5 weeks.

When the orientation process has been completed, the principal and the school staff meet to review testing results and prior school history in order to plan a schedule. All residents are on "new boy" status during this time and are not allowed weekend passes, although family members can visit on the weekends. In general, the orientation period is a time of active planning by the different departments to evaluate a particular youngster's educational and treatment needs. The social services department develops a formal written initial treatment plan and the school develops an individual educational plan. During this time, the program solicits relevant information from prior treatment and educational experiences, such as school transcripts, hospital discharge summaries, outpatient treatment summaries, and any prior psychological and/or educational evaluations.

CONCLUSIONS

Although Ocean Tides started years before what is now referred to as "positive psychology" had its influence on the field of behavioral health, the program was ahead of its time in its philosophy that the way to help troubled youngsters was to identify and build on their strengths. This approach contrasted sharply with the "deficit" model of juvenile delinquency that was prevalent when the program began. The prevailing belief in this model is that troubled youngsters are "broken" and in need of repair. At Ocean Tides, a positive orientation is used in a variety of specific ways in the program to rehabilitate the residents. Many of these specific policies and practices developed gradually over time from staff discussions, brainstorming, soul searching, problem solving, and trial-and-error approaches. In this process, outside consultants have been used to provide occasional input in the form of workshops or ongoing consultation to the staff to help them develop, innovate, and make changes to the program. In the next chapter, the authors describe how the role of the consultant can be used to help shape the development and maintenance of a program.

REFERENCES

Agnew, R. (2005). *Why do criminals offend? A general theory of crime and delinquency.* Los Angeles, CA: Roxbury.

Alexander, J. F., & Parsons, B. V. (1973). Short-term behavioral intervention with delinquent families: Impact on family process and recidivism. *Journal of Abnormal Psychology, 81*(3), 219–225.

Alexander, J. F., Waldron, H. B., Robbins, M. S., & Neeb, A. A. (2013). *Functional family therapy for adolescent behavior problems.* Washington, DC: American Psychological Association.

Beachaine, T. P., Hinshaw, S. P., & Pang, K. L. (2010). Comorbidity of attention-deficit/hyperactivity disorder and early-onset hyperactivity disorder and early-onset conduct disorder: Biological, environmental, and developmental mechanisms. *Clinical Psychology, 17*, 327–336.

Glasser, W. (1965). *Reality therapy: A new approach to psychiatry.* New York, NY: Harper & Row.

Grebstein, L. C. (1986). An eclectic family therapy. In J. Norcross (Ed.), *Handbook of eclectic psychotherapy* (pp. 282–319). New York, NY: Brunner/Mazel.

Greenwood, P. W. (2006). *Changing lives: Delinquency prevention as crime control policy.* Chicago, IL: University of Chicago Press.

Guerra, N. G., Kim, T. E., & Boxer, P. (2008). What works: Best practices for juvenile offenders. In R. D. Hoge, N. G. Guerra, & P. Boxer (Eds.), *Treating the juvenile offender* (pp. 79–102). New York, NY: Guilford Press.

Haley, J. (1972). *Strategies of psychotherapy.* New York, NY: Grune & Stratton.

Haley, J. (1976). *Problem-solving therapy.* San Francisco, CA: Jossey-Bass.

Haley, J., & Hoffman, L. (1967). *Techniques of family therapy.* New York, NY: Basic Books.

Hengeller, S. W., Schoenwald, S. K., Borduin, C. M., Rowland, M. D., & Cunningham, P. B. (1998). *Multisystemic treatment of antisocial behavior in children and adolescents.* New York, NY: Guilford Press.

Lerner, R. M. (2005). *Promoting positive youth development: Theoretical and empirical bases.* White paper prepared for Workshop on the Science of Adolescent

Health and Development, National Research Council, Washington, DC. National Research Council/Institute of Medicine. Washington, DC: National Academy of Sciences. Retrieved from ase.tufts.edu/iaryd/documents/pubpromotingpositive.pdf

Loes, A., & Huether, F. (Eds.). (1994). *Meditations by John Baptist de La Salle.* Landover, MD: Christian Brothers Conference.

Minuchin, S. (1974). *Families and family therapy.* Cambridge, MA: Harvard University Press.

Minuchin, S., & Fishman, H. C. (1981). *Family therapy techniques.* Cambridge, MA: Harvard University Press.

Ocean Tides. (1980). *Handbook for school staff.* Narrragansett, RI: Author.

Ocean Tides. (1988). *Social services department handbook.* Narragansett, RI: Author.

Ocean Tides. (2011). *Group living staff handbook.* Narragansett, RI: Author.

Plomin, R. H., Chipuer, M., & Lochlin, J. C. (1990). Behavioral genetics and personality. In L. A. Pervin (Ed.), *Handbook of personality theory and research* (pp. 225–243). New York, NY: Guilford Press.

Rhodes, J. E. (2002). *Stand by me: The risks and rewards of mentoring today's youth.* Cambridge, MA: Harvard University Press.

Romig, D. A. (1978). *Justice for our children.* Lexington, MA: D. C. Heath.

Sexton, T., & Turner, C. W. (2010). The effectiveness of functional family therapy for youth with behavioral problems in a community practice setting. *Journal of Family Psychology, 24*(3), 339–348.

Shoemaker, D. J. (2009). *Juvenile delinquency.* Lanham, MD: Rowman & Littlefield.

CHAPTER 7

Navigating the Waters: The Role of the Clinical Psychologist as a Consultant

The role of the consultant in programs for juveniles is important to help shape its development and maintenance. This is especially significant when the program is grounded in positive psychology, at identifying and further developing programmatic and individual-level strengths in its participants. Our goal in this chapter is to describe how consultants from clinical psychology and social work can be used in a residential rehabilitation program for male juvenile delinquents. Most consultants are used for relatively short periods of time to provide specific types of services. This is true at Ocean Tides and this use of consultants is described later in this chapter and at other places in the book. The main focus is on the long-term use of a single consultant and how the nature of consultation is a reciprocal process. That is, while a consultant provides advice and other services, interacting with the delinquents and the staff provides the consultant with valuable knowledge and insights that enhance and improve the nature of the consultation. Viewed in this context, consultation works as a feedback loop. What is unusual in this situation is that the same consultant has remained with the program since its inception. This type of long-term consultation requires a consultant to evolve, change, and adapt as the program grows and develops.

DEFINING THE ROLE OF THE CONSULTANT

The use of the term "consultant" varies considerably in human service agencies. In some cases, it is used to refer to professionals from outside the agency who are hired on a part-time basis to provide direct professional services, such as psychotherapy or diagnostic psychological testing, to the agency's clients. Although the title "consultant" is often used to describe this role, the position would be more accurately described as a part-time clinician. In this chapter, the use of the term "consultant" follows Caplan's (1970) definition of the consultant as a specialist who is enlisted by an agency or program to get help with a current work problem that is presenting some difficulty. In describing the functions of the consultant, Caplan (1970) further restricts his definition to indicate that the professional responsibility for the services provided to the clients remains with the organization, not the consultant.

> The consultant may offer helpful clarifications, diagnostic formulations, or advice on treatment; but the consultee will be free to accept or reject all or part of the help . . . Another essential aspect of this type of consultation is that the consultant engages in the activity not only in order to help the consultee with his current work problem in relation to a specific client or program but also in order to add to the consultee's knowledge and to lessen areas of misunderstanding, so that he may be able in the future to deal more effectively on his own with this category of problem. (Caplan, 1970, p. 20)

The role of the consultant at Ocean Tides is very much in keeping with Caplan's (1970) definition of a consultant in that his primary role is to offer technical assistance and emotional support to the staff, rather than to provide direct services to the residents. Any direct services the consultant provides has to have at least one staff member present as an observer so that the consultant can serve as a role model for training purposes. There are only a few exceptions to this model: undergraduate student interns and regular staff members occasionally sit in on the interviews as observers and for training; and at the nonresidential satellite campus of Ocean Tides School where the consultant provides both assessment and short-term counseling to selected students.

PHILOSOPHY OF CONSULTATION

The basic philosophy of consultation is that the consultant is like a guide in mountain climbing. The guide advises on the choice of the route, the pace of climbing, what equipment is needed, the best time to go, and other relevant information. However, the client does the climbing and the hiking. If the client gets tired and cannot go on, he or she can rest. The guide does not carry the client or provide "piggyback" service. Hence it is with the role of the consultant. In this view of consultation, the success of the program is directly related to the quality of the staff. The primary role of the consultant is to help the staff develop and utilize their skills and talents to a higher level: positive psychology.

As staff members have the most contact with the residents of a program, they know the residents better than an outside consultant, who has more limited contact. In mental hospitals, the nurses and mental health workers who are on the wards usually know the patients better than psychiatrists, psychologists, or social workers, who may have only occasional and limited contact with the patients. The failure to regularly check with full-time staff about the behavior of the residents can have serious consequences. The following anecdote vividly describes the kind of mistake or inaccurate assumption that can result from not consulting with residential staff.

An intern at a large Veterans Affairs hospital for psychiatric patients volunteered to lead a new group on one of the locked wards for committed, actively suicidal, or otherwise dangerous patients. Prior to starting the group, his supervisor told him that one of the patients in the group (Mr. F) was legally committed because of paranoid schizophrenia. The supervisor then challenged the intern to find any evidence of psychosis or, in fact, any evidence of abnormal thinking or behavior of any kind. The intern's first impression of Mr. F was that he was very bright, articulate, and persuasive. The only indication of any possible disturbance was that he frequently was unkempt in his grooming and came to the group without having shaved or combed his hair. There were no indications of irrational or unusual thinking or behavior.

As the group unfolded, Mr. F emerged as the dominant member of the group and regularly monopolized the sessions. The other patients were more than happy to oblige and let him do all the talking. He told the same story over and over again. He said that this was his second time in the hospital. The first time he had come in, he had in fact been psychotic but did not recognize it or acknowledge it. It took him 2 years under the excellent care of Dr. B, his psychiatrist, to get better enough to leave the hospital. He was discharged after several trial visits and had been out of the hospital and doing well for more than a year. Then he started to "slip." Unlike the first time, he noticed the symptoms early and checked himself in before he got worse. That was his big mistake. In the time he was out, Dr. B was no longer his ward psychiatrist, having moved up to an administrative position, and the hospital had "changed for the worse" in his opinion. Consequently, he tried to "elope" (run away). As a result, Mr. F's uncle had him legally committed and himself appointed legal guardian by the court. Mr. F alleged that his uncle did this so that he could gain control of Mr. F's money (he had a substantial service-connected disability pension). Mr. F argued that he had not been psychotic at the time of his readmission, but that if he was now it was because of his experiences in the hospital. He complained of being on a ward with very disturbed patients who did not care for themselves. They often soiled themselves, spit and urinated on the floor, and, in general, were difficult to be around. He only had 1 hour a day that he was allowed to be outside. Mr. F would repeatedly challenge the group leader by stating: "You stay around people like that every day and all day long and see how long you stay sane! If I wasn't crazy when I got here, I probably am now." He also had a history of frequent attempted elopements, which is why he remained on a locked ward. When the intern tried to point out to the patient that he would probably be transferred to a non locked ward if he would stop trying to run away, the patient always had a logical rejoinder that he had tried that and it did not do any good. Although it was frustrating to deal with him and listen to him go over the same story repeatedly, he did not show any signs of psychosis or schizophrenia.

One day a new patient joined the group who was on the locked ward because he had made a serious suicide attempt prior to coming to the hospital. He was obviously depressed and did not say much in the group. After several meetings, he finally spoke up shortly after one of Mr. F's tirades. He mildly and somewhat timidly commented that he had only been in the hospital for a few weeks, but that he noticed that only one patient on the ward spit and urinated on floor and that was Mr. F! The normally composed and articulate Mr. F responded immediately by jumping up and launching into a wild, disorganized, and blatantly psychotic verbal attack directed at his accuser. He ranted and raved about how he had been victimized by aliens sent to purposely destroy his mind and a variety of other equally bizarre accusations.

The point of this story is that the intern had not checked with either the ward nurses or mental health workers to find out if there was any truth in Mr. F's attributions and complaints. His naive stereotyping of severe mental illness had prevented him from perceiving the true nature of the patient's difficulties. In dealing with delinquents who routinely lie, externalize the responsibility for and blame others for their problems, and allege various kinds of verbal and abuse by the staff, it is essential to check patients' or residents' stories with relevant staff.

The Changing Role of the Consultant Over Time

The role of the consultant changes as an organization changes and grows. In the early stages a program's development, much of the consultant's time is spent in providing in-service training and feedback to a small and relatively inexperienced staff. For example, when Ocean Tides first began, the consultant met weekly with each of the three staff components of the program: the teachers, social workers, and group-living staff. The specific nature of these meetings and training varied with the type of staff. In working with the group-living (residential) staff, the consultant's primary role involved training the staff in specific skills in how to deal with the residents, particularly when they were upset. With the teachers, consultation involved helping them develop effective procedures for discipline, dealing with difficult youngsters in the classroom, and creating alternative methods of instruction. In meeting with the social services staff, discussion of particular cases and specific methods of intervention, such as family therapy techniques, was the focus. Regardless of the specific nature of the consultation, the primary focus was to encourage the staff to brainstorm and take the initiative in developing their ideas and procedures.

As suggested by the anecdote described earlier, it is important to have direct knowledge about the residents to be able to provide effective consultation and training to the staff. In the early days of the program, some of the most useful time the consultant spent was in observing staff members' interactions with the residents. Visiting in the evenings while the residents were watching TV or engaged in other leisure time activities was particularly helpful. In addition to getting to know the residents better, this allowed the consultant to directly observe staff interactions in an in unobtrusive manner. These observations were invaluable in discussing situations in his meetings with staff when there were discrepancies between what a staff member reported about an interaction with a resident and what the consultant had observed. Similarly, in working with teachers, having direct classroom observations is essential. With social workers, the consultant was available to occasionally sit in on an individual counseling session or a family meeting if the social worker felt that he or she wanted an independent opinion.

SPECIFIC FUNCTIONS OF THE CONSULTANT

The role of the consultant over the years has involved all of Caplan's (1970) four types of mental health consultation: client-centered case consultation, consultee-centered case consultation, program-centered administrative consultation, and consultee-centered administrative consultation. *Client-centered case consultation* involves using specialized skills and knowledge to determine the nature of the problem and make specific recommendation on how to deal with the case. In *consultee-centered case consultation,* the goal is also to help the client deal more effectively with the case, but the emphasis is on the client's difficulty in dealing with the case. *Program-centered case consultation* involves developing new programs and improving existing ones. *Consultee-centered administrative consultation* involves helping the administrators of a program identify and improve difficulties in development, organization, and implementation of policies and procedures.

The specific functions of the consultant are many, varied, and continually changing. These duties include providing emotional support to staff, both collectively and with individual staff members; technical support (e.g., in-service training in specific procedures, such as family therapy techniques); along with other consultants, meet monthly with the social services staff to discuss difficult cases; conflict mediation and resolution when staff have disagreements; identifying problems and guiding problem-solving discussions; leading and moderating full staff meetings about program development and related issues; acting as a mediator between staff and administration regarding grievances and dissatisfactions; developing procedures for evaluation of staff and administrators; and conducting annual evaluations of department heads and administrators with accompanying written reports.

Emotional Support of Staff

Research on psychotherapy has consistently reaffirmed the importance of the therapeutic relationship as an essential ingredient for positive outcomes. Key components of this relationship are trust, empathy, and support. Working with troubled youngsters is emotionally demanding, stressful, and often frustrating. Consequently, it can be difficult for staff members to maintain a positive attitude. If staff and teachers are to be effective, they need to monitor their reactions and keep their own emotional house in order. One of the unique aspects of the Ocean Tides program is its attendance to the emotional welfare of the staff as well as the residents. Since the program began, one of the main and most important aspects of the consultant's role has been to help create a work environment that provides ongoing emotional support to the staff. For example, in his weekly meetings with the teachers, the consultant encourages them to share and discuss not only their problems with residents but their frustrations, feelings of helplessness, anger, discouragement, and other negative feelings. The consultant's goals for meetings with the residential staff are similar to those with the teachers. Encouraging staff to express their feelings about their work is more easily said than done. Teachers and residential staff are not used to publicly sharing their personal frustrations and other negative emotions. Sometimes they are unwilling to even acknowledge these feelings to themselves. It requires considerable patience, tact, and skill on the part of the consultant to create an atmosphere in which teachers and other staff members felt safe enough to candidly discuss their true feelings.

In order to accomplish these goals, a consultant occasionally uses other materials. For example, in the early days of the program, when the size of the staff was much smaller, the consultant recommended the staff to read an interesting book by Grossman (1972), *Nine Rotten Lousy Kids*, as a way of giving them permission to talk honestly about their feelings. This fascinating book tells the story of an experimental school in New York City for delinquent boys and "nine of the kids who attended that school instead of the state training schools, mental hospitals and residential treatment centers the courts had already assigned them to." The school was based on the belief that these youngsters could be helped "not by punishing them for their problems or removing them far from the communities they know, but rather by understanding the conditions that caused their difficulties and by answering their hopelessness with optimism, their alienation with friendship, their suspiciousness with trust, and their anger with love" (Grossman, 1972, p. vii). The book is based on a daily log dictated by the staff of what happened, how it happened, and the thoughts and feelings of the staff. Despite its title, which might suggest that the staff held a negative view of the youngsters and their work with them, it is an honest and uncensored account of what it is like to work with difficult youngsters. The book provides an excellent model for staff to discuss their experiences with candor and openness.

Conducting Workshops and In-Service Training

Success in communicating with these young men requires understanding, patience, tact, skill in communicating, and knowledge of oneself. The consultants conduct workshops with staff that provide suggestions and guidelines. The goals of these workshops are to provide basic information that will be useful in the staff's interactions with the residents; to provide specialized knowledge for dealing with specific types of situations; and to have the ideas serve as a point of departure for discussion. Some examples of ideas presented at workshops are described in the following:

Know Thyself

The first step in trying to help others is to be aware of one's own personality and state of mind at the time one is interacting with another person. All of us have "bad days" or maybe even bad hours or minutes. At these times, we are likely to be irritable, less patient, or less tolerant of behaviors that would ordinarily not bother us. Consequently, we may overreact or respond in ways that are not helpful. One of the few characteristics that the residents have in common is that they have all had to learn how to survive in difficult circumstances. One of the most popular survival skills used by adolescents in dealing with adults is to find some vulnerability in the adult and attack it. The basic strategy is that the best defense is a good offense.

Many of the residents at Ocean Tides have considerable street smarts and have developed this strategy into an art form. They are masters at knowing how to provoke or bait staff into saying or doing things that they might later regret. An effective antidote to this behavior is for staff to be aware of their own vulnerability so that they are not surprised or caught off guard. Simple things, such as not having a good night's sleep, being worried or preoccupied about personal issues, or not feeling well physically, can make staff more susceptible to reacting inappropriately to the residents or each other. When staff members come to work, it is important for them to be aware of their state of mind and to take that into consideration in dealing with the youngsters. Some examples of common feelings a staff member might experience in dealing with the residents include exhaustion, ineffectiveness, anger, frustration, disgust, feeling disrespected, insecurity, burnout, apathy, and loss of control. These feelings, if not recognized and dealt with, can lead to inappropriate and ineffective responses, including overreacting by premature or too harsh discipline, provocative behavior that escalates rather than diffuses a situation, and inappropriate verbal responses.

Understand the Residents

The Ocean Tides residents represent a wide range of individual differences in their personalities; intelligence and cognitive abilities; and socioeconomic, ethnic, and racial backgrounds. In recent years, the types of young men who end up in the juvenile justice system, and consequently at Ocean Tides, are considerably more complex than in the earlier days of the program. Many of them have been in the mental health system and are genuinely emotionally disturbed. Almost all of them have very low self-esteem; strong feelings of insecurity; and are used to failure, neglect, abuse, rejection, abandonment, and disrespect from others, particularly adults. The task in attempting to rehabilitate these young men is to establish an emotionally positive environment in which negative attitudes are replaced by more positive feelings. It is important to remember that there is no one right way of dealing with the residents or of responding to a situation. In fact, there are times when even the most experienced staff member may find it difficult to know how to respond because of the behavior of the resident or the complexity of the situation. A good principle to remember is that no one size fits all. Each resident is a unique individual requiring an individualized response and every situation is different. What might work one time with a resident might not work again in a similar situation with the same resident.

The Use of Reframing

One of the techniques used in teaching staff to help the residents change their negative ideas and related behavior is "reframing." Therapists often use this technique to try to find positive aspects of what on the surface appear to be negative thoughts or behaviors. This can be very useful for understanding the underlying motivation for negative behavior, for using that understanding to defuse a potentially difficult situation, and for redirecting the behavior. Listed here are some examples of "reframes" of difficult and negative behaviors that are common among our residents. Some of these reframes have been adapted from Appelstein (1998).

NEGATIVE LABEL	MORE POSITIVE REFRAME
Manipulative	Good at controlling the situation and getting needs met
Stubborn and defiant	Assertive and good at standing up for yourself
Obnoxious	Good at pushing people away and being left alone
Tantrum or outburst	Good at getting someone to pay attention
Won't talk	Loyalty to friends or family
Resistant	Cautious
Foul mouthed	Expressive
Silly and disruptive	A creative person

There are several good reasons to look for positive elements in negative behaviors: (a) The staff member is more likely to respond differently and in a more helpful way; (b) by pointing out the positive element, it often catches the resident by surprise and allows a staff member to defuse or otherwise alter a potentially difficult situation; and (c) it helps to establish and maintain a more positive and trusting relationship with the resident.

Training Staff to Deal With Difficult Residents

Another important topic used in training staff is how to deal with difficult residents. Difficult residents are youngsters who act in one or more of the following ways: They are actively or overtly aggressive (including insulting, threatening, hostile sounding, sarcastic, or condescending); passive-aggressive (instead of admitting that they are upset, they pout, refuse to talk, or engage in the "silent treatment"); stubborn and argumentative; critical and judgmental; lie or intentionally distort or misrepresent their behavior or situations; unintentionally distort situations; and chronically complain.

Dealing with a youngster who is hostile or aggressive is one of the most common and difficult situations. A good way to try and defuse anger is to listen to the resident, acknowledge his anger, and point out the hostile way he is expressing it. A resident has a right to feel angry but not to express it in any way he wants. Letting the resident know (in a calm and matter-of-fact manner) that the way he is expressing his anger is inappropriate can help calm the waters. By drawing attention to how the staff member is being treated helps change the focus. It is important to emphasize that this will not work with residents who are enraged, out of control, or irrational. When this occurs, the focus shifts to crisis intervention with the goal of keeping the situation from escalating. When a resident is upset to the point of being out of control, almost any response will probably provoke him further or escalate the situation. In these instances, the most important objective is to allow the person to calm down.

It is not uncommon for adolescents to respond to adults by giving them the silent treatment, particularly when they are angry or upset. When this occurs, it is important to try to empathize with the resident. Instead of insisting that he talk, ask in a genuine and friendly way why he does not want to talk to you. If that does not work, suggest that this may not be a good time and suggest that he can talk things over later when he is more in the mood. The essential point is to avoid getting into a power struggle. The youngster may want to be combative. Try not to take the bait. It is important that staff members or teachers do not deal with a youngster when he is upset or angry. Responding out of anger increases the probability of saying or doing something that might make matters worse. Except in genuine crisis situations, the staff member has plenty of time to deal with the youngster when they both are calmer.

Instead of clamming up, sometimes residents are argumentative. Although it is natural to focus on his behavior, an effective alternative is to listen more carefully. Burns (1989) describes five techniques for effective communication, including three listening skills and two self-expression skills to deal with difficult situations. The listening skills include (a) *the disarming technique* in which one tries to find some truth in what the youngster is saying, even if one thinks that what he is saying is totally wrong, unreasonable, irrational, or unfair; (b) *empathy*, in which one tries to see things from the other person's perspective; and (c) *inquiry*, which involves asking gentle, probing questions to learn more about what the youngster is thinking and feeling. Self-expression skills involve *stroking* and *"I feel"* statements. *Stroking* is when a staff member tries to find something genuinely positive to say to the resident, even in the heat of battle. This strategy communicates respect and can help cool down a hot situation. *"I feel"* statements involve making "I" rather than "you" statements. For example, "I feel upset when you..." or "I don't like it when..." instead of "You're wrong!" or "You're making me mad" (Burns, 1989, p. 419).

It is important to not patronize a youngster or give him the impression that he is not being taken seriously. Genuineness is essential for effective communication. It is also important to remember that there are some residents with whom it may not be possible to communicate, either at particular times or in general, although this is rare. As the saying goes, "There is no arguing with a closed mind." It is essential that it is not the staff member's mind that is the one that is closed.

Many of the residents have significant issues with power and control. They want to have their own way and have often been successful in defying authority figures in the past, such as parents and teachers. Although the program is structured and has clear rules, residents are likely to challenge the rules in general or the authority of a particular staff member. This can be one of the most trying issues to deal with and requires tact, patience, and keeping cool. Some suggestions for the effective use of power that have been presented in in-service training workshops include the following:

1. Do not abuse or misuse your power by being authoritarian, arbitrary, unfair, or unilateral. Make sure that you know and understand the program's rules.
2. Do not discipline out of anger or frustration.
3. Before disciplining a youngster, *warn* him about possible consequences. Focus on his behavior and make sure (usually by asking) if he is aware that he is doing something wrong or acting inappropriately.

4. Whenever possible, try to empower the residents to solve his own problems. Ask what he would do or what he thinks are appropriate consequences (you do not have to agree with them or follow their recommendations).
5. Give residents reasons for your response or sanction. They have a right to an explanation. If they "play dumb" or keep asking why, you can always indicate that you explained. They have a right to disagree or be upset.
6. Avoid authoritarian pronouncements like "Because I told you so!" or "Because I said so!"
7. When in doubt about how to handle a situation or you recognize that you are upset, do nothing! You can always decide on a suitable response later when you are calmer or have had a chance to consult with a colleague. It is appropriate and effective to tell a resident that there will be consequences but you want to think about it before you decide.
8. Do not say or do anything to a youngster that you would not want said or done to you. Remember, the main way in which children learn is by modeling or imitating the behavior of adults. Act in the ways that you want them to act. They are very sensitive to discrepancies in your words and behaviors.
9. Make sure your discipline is appropriate to the offense. Be consistent with the same youngster and with different youngsters.
10. Treat the residents with respect. This is a key issue for them. Even though they treat others disrespectfully, they expect to be treated with respect. Use words like *please* and *thank you* in your interactions. According to Gilligan (1997), perceived disrespect is a key factor in causing violent behavior. He notes:

> [T]he prison inmates I work with have told me repeatedly, when I asked them why they had assaulted someone, that it was because "he disrespected me," or "he disrespected my visit" (meaning "visitor"). The word "disrespect" is so central in the vocabulary, moral value system, and psychodynamics of these chronically violent men that they have abbreviated it into the slang term, "he dis'ed me." (Gilligan, 1997, pp. 105–106)

Behaviors for Staff to Avoid

There are certain behaviors that staff members should always avoid in dealing with the residents. These include never using insulting, hostile, sarcastic, or condescending language even if it is meant as a joke. Do not mock a youngster, call him names, tease him, or taunt him. No matter how angry or frustrated you may feel, do not regress to a resident's level of behavior. Once you have established a good working relationship with mutual trust, good-natured teasing and playfulness are natural. Be careful. Many residents have impulse control problems or short fuses and what appears to be a playful situation can very quickly (and without warning) change and escalate into a difficult encounter. Avoiding physical contact or direct confrontation is important. On rare instances, it may be necessary to restrain a youngster to prevent or break up a fight. If this is necessary, get help from other staff. Ocean Tides is not a program that uses restraints. If a youngster gets out of control and starts throwing things, leave him alone. Physical objects can be replaced. Positive reinforcement is a useful alternative to punishment and can also be used to establish and maintain better relationships with a youngster.

No set of guidelines is a substitute for good judgment and common sense. All of the aforementioned suggestions are not intended to create a robot-like or automatic set of responses by staff to the residents. Every staff member has his or her own unique style and personality and should feel free to use those in interacting with the residents. Working with delinquent youngsters is an ongoing work in progress, in which staff members try to learn from their mistakes.

Conflict Mediation and Resolution

An important function of the role of a consultant is to mediate the occasional conflicts that arise among staff. Sometimes they occur between staff members in different departments, who, by virtue of their different responsibilities and relationships with the residents, disagree about how to respond to the residents. This is particularly true with regard to discipline. For example, teachers and residential counselors may differ in how and when to discipline or use sanctions, either with regard to the type of behavior involved or the leniency or harshness of the sanction.

This particular disagreement is reminiscent of the good parent–bad parent arguments that occur within families.

Sometimes there are significant differences of opinion between members of the same department. In the early days of the program, when policies and procedures were still in development, there were major differences of opinion among teachers with regard to acceptable behavior in the classroom and appropriate disciplinary procedures. In the residential part of the program, staff who share a shift may feel that one or the other is "not carrying his or her weight," not supervising the residents closely enough, or is being too lax in terms of sanctioning inappropriate behavior. The consultant serves as mediator in these disputes with the task of not only helping the involved parties reach some sort of compromise or working solution but also helping them maintain mutual respect and the ability to continue to work together in a cooperative, mutually supportive, and cohesive manner.

Finally, a whole variety of issues can develop between the administrators and the staff. These are similar to the classic labor–management disputes regarding productivity, compensation, being appreciated, and trust. Again, the consultants have the task of being aware of these problems as they arise and finding ways to help resolve them. One important function of the consultant is to present concerns that the staff has to the administration. This is always done with the advance knowledge and consent of the staff. For the consultant to be able to serve as a successful mediator between staff and administration, he or she must have the complete trust of both parties.

Identifying Problems and Guiding Problem-Solving Discussions

A major task of any consultant is to provide a "fresh pair of eyes" so to speak—to examine the program and note inconsistencies, policies that are not working, and other problems. Perhaps the best way to illustrate this type of consultation is to describe a specific example having to do with weekend activities. The problem identified by the residential staff was that residents who had failed to earn weekend passes (or "lost their weekends") because of behavior problems did not appear to change their behavior for the better. Losing a weekend pass to go home is the ultimate sanction and occurs only after an accumulation of violations.

The residential aspect of the program has a graded disciplinary procedure in which residents are given "time" (time-outs) for misbehavior. As the amount of time accumulates, it can result in partial or total loss of the weekend pass to home. Some youngsters remain in residence for the weekend for non disciplinary reason. They are on new resident orientation (first 5 weeks in the program) or have no acceptable pass resource. These residents go to the movies, local sporting events, go swimming at a local university pool, visit the nearby beach in the summer, and participate in other enjoyable supervised recreational activities.

The problem was that the youngsters who lost their weekends for disciplinary reasons participated in the same activities and received the same privileges as residents still on orientation or who did not have suitable family with which to visit during weekends. Instead of being perceived as discipline for unacceptable behavior, the loss of the weekend pass could be interpreted by the residents as a reward for negative behavior. In this instance, the consultant initiated a discussion with the staff about alternative activities on the weekend that would be both beneficial to the program and not considered a reward. The staff brainstormed and came up with the notion of doing "housework" (cleaning). Although there was general agreement that this was a good idea, as with all changes, there was some initial resistance. If some of the residents were involved in activities and other residents had to do housework, this meant additional supervisory responsibility for staff as well as having to deal the complaints from some of the residents of unfairness and differential treatment. The change was implemented with positive results and remains in place as a part of the program.

Leading and Moderating Staff Meetings

For any treatment program to be successful, it is essential that there is good communication at all levels. An effective consultant can play a major role in ensuring that there is good communication by helping to devise and implement procedures that will facilitate good communication. The first step is to convince the top administrator that good communication within and between departments and program components is important and to obtain his or her support. The most efficient way of accomplishing good communication is through regular staff meetings on at least a weekly but preferably daily basis. The meetings can be short but should include information that staff members need to know. For example, is a resident having a bad day or have any extraordinary events or situations occurred in the past 24 hours that might affect a resident's behavior?

In the early stage of a program's development, the consultant can play a major role in facilitating staff meetings in which policy and procedures are being developed. There are often differences of opinion with regard to these issues. A good facilitator can help resolve these differences in ways that will lead to positive outcomes. Once procedures are in place, it is important to periodically review them to see if they continue to be effective and are in keeping with the goals and values of the program. As an outside observer, the consultant can play a major role in eliciting open and honest discussion regarding dissatisfactions with the program and resolving interdepartmental and intradepartmental differences of opinion with regard to both the philosophy and practical applications of treatment.

As a clinical psychologist with a family systems orientation, the consultant tends to view the world and its organizations in family terms. It is not unusual at full staff meetings, where all the program's staff members are present, for sibling rivalry issues to erupt and for various administrators to adopt roles as parent or grandparent surrogates. For example, staff members of one department may feel that they work harder, or know the kids better, or have more effective ways of dealing with the residents. Sometimes these opinions are expressed in the form of criticism of other departments. Department heads may respond as indulgent parents who are protective of their children and make excuses for their behavior. It is important for the consultant to be able to monitor and mediate these disputes. At other times, problems have to do with staff members feeling undervalued, overworked, or underpaid. Again, it is important for these issues to be brought out in the open and addressed directly.

Development of the Family Program

One of the consultant's most important contributions to the program has been the introduction of the importance of working with the boys' families while they are in residence. The establishment of the Ocean Tides program in the mid-1970s coincided with the emergence of family systems and communications theories of psychopathology. These approaches put less emphasis on the intrapsychic causes of symptomatic behavior characteristic of psychodynamic approaches and focused more on the relational and communication patterns in the family as the main determinants of problem behavior. Although a particular person in the family might emerge as the symptom bearer or "identified patient," it was the family that was the focus for treatment. As family therapy evolved, the view expanded from perceiving the family as being the cause of individual symptoms to seeing the family as affected by problem behavior.

As none of the staff had any experience with family therapy, there was initial resistance to the idea that it was important to work with the families of the boys while they were in residence. Many staff members believed that the families were too dysfunctional and were not amenable to counseling. What was needed was an "ice breaker." After much discussion, the staff agreed to invite the families of the residents to come to Ocean Tides to see the facilities where their sons would be staying, to gather together in the dining room for light refreshments, and to meet the staff. Contrary to the dire predictions of many of the staff that few, if any, family members would show up, every resident had at least one parent or representative family member attending this initial meeting. Shortly after this meeting, the consultant initiated in-service training in family therapy for the social services staff.

Most of the families of these boys are not well suited for traditional family therapy. Nevertheless, it is important to work with the families to help create a better environment for the boys to return to following completion of the program and to improve their relationships within the family. The family counseling approach used at Ocean Tides is an eclectic model (Grebstein, 1986) that utilizes aspects of structural family therapy (Minuchin, 1974; Minuchin & Fishman, 1981); strategic family therapy (Haley, 1972, 1976); and problem-centered systems therapy of the family (Epstein & Bishop, 1981). Social services counselors are trained in how to assess a family by taking a three-generational family history using a genogram (Guerin & Pendagast, 1976) and assessing six areas of family function as described in the McMaster model (Epstein, Bishop, & Levin, 1978). This model identifies these basic functions, such as: *problem solving* (the family's usual way of resolving both instrumental or task-oriented and feeling-related problems); *communication* (the family's style of exchanging information); *affective responsiveness* (the capacity of the family members to respond emotionally to each other); *affective involvement* (the extent to which family members value, care for, or show interest in each other); *behavior control* (the methods a family applies for monitoring the behavior of its members, i.e., discipline); and *roles* (the repeating patterns of behavior that individuals use to fulfill family functions). These particular dimensions of family behavior came out of a study of nonclinical families (Epstein, Sigal, & Rakoff, 1962). Family counseling has limited goals and focuses on trying to improve communication, parental control and discipline, and the expression of positive feelings and caring. Different consultants in clinical psychology and clinical social work with expertise in family therapy provide ongoing case consultation with the social services department.

Development of Evaluation Procedures

The consultant provides two types of evaluations. One type is a clinical psychological evaluation of referred residents. These evaluations are primarily done by interview and are described in detail in the following chapter on interviewing delinquents. The other evaluations are annual evaluations of program administrators, typically the department heads. These evaluations are done annually and consist of both a group interview format and a rating form that is completed anonymously. The evaluation form is included in Appendix B and the actual process of conducting the evaluations is described in the next section.

Conducting Annual Evaluations of Administrators

The procedure for conducting an evaluation of an administrator or head of a department consists of two parts. In the first part, all members of a particular department (i.e., teachers, residential staff, social workers, or group home staff) individually and anonymously complete the 20-item performance evaluation form with the opportunity to add written comments. The results of the evaluation form are summarized in both actual number and percent in a written report. Any additional written comments are included verbatim. The second part of the evaluation report contains a summary of additional comments regarding the administrator's job performance that were obtained using a structured group interview. These comments are organized into the following three categories: administrative skills; supervisory skills and staff relations; and relations with residents. After the interview, the consultant integrates the comments into a descriptive report and makes a draft copy of the report available to the involved staff for their corrections and approval. Once the staff agrees that the report accurately reflects their views, a final report is submitted to the director of the program. The director then goes over the evaluation with the administrator under review.

Generally, the evaluation process goes smoothly to the extent that people participate and are sincere and candid in their appraisal. Some of the problems that have occurred include doubts about the real anonymity of the feedback. Some staff members have indicated that they are reluctant to express themselves candidly out of concern that any unfavorable comments might be traced back to them. Occasionally, a staff member will respond to the rating form with no variation in rankings. For example, the rating form will be completed with every item checked as "excellent" or "poor." When this occurs, the consultant usually interprets this response as "going through the motions" or not taking the evaluation seriously and will comment on this in his report.

Other Roles of the Consultant

Sometimes it is necessary to hire consultants with special expertise for specific roles. They are used in three ways. They may provide ongoing services, such as devising and leading special programs, namely the sexual offender program or substance abuse group. In these cases, they colead groups with a regular staff member. A second way in which a consultant may be used is to present a workshop or in-service training of staff members. This is usually a single event rather than an ongoing activity. The third use of the consultant can involve ongoing in-service with a particular department. For example, the social services department has a monthly in-service with an outside consultant in social work who is a former faculty member at a local school of social work.

CONCLUSIONS

Defining and explaining the roles played by a clinical psychologist working as a consultant to a program like Ocean Tides are difficult because it is the epitome of multitasking and those roles shift and mold to conform to changing needs. It is not necessary that all of these roles are played by the same consultant, but it is very important that they share a common philosophy and that they regularly communicate with one another. Ocean Tides operates in much the same way as a family does, and if two parents have divergent ideas about how to raise their children, then conflict ensues. Communication is the key to a successful program—among administrators, staff, teachers, residents, and everyone who is involved. This goal is accomplished best by intermediaries who are trained and skilled at facilitating this kind of communication—those who understand the needs of staff, teachers, administrators, and residents. The consultant, whether he or she is a clinical psychologist, clinical social worker, or other specialist in behavioral health, thus plays an integral role in rehabilitating juvenile offenders before he or she ever even interacts directly with the residents.

REFERENCES

Appelstein, C. (1998). *No such thing as a bad kid.* Weston, MA: Gifford School.

Burns, D. D. (1989). *The feeling good handbook.* New York, NY: William Morrow.

Caplan, G. (1970). *The theory and practice of mental health consultation.* New York, NY: Basic Books.

Epstein, N. B., & Bishop, D. S. (1981). Problem-centered systems therapy of the family. In A. S. Gurman & D. P. Kniskern (Eds.), *Handbook of family therapy* (pp. 444–482). New York, NY: Brunner/Mazel.

Epstein, N. B., Bishop, D. S., & Levin, S. (1978). The McMaster model of family functioning. *Journal of Marriage and Family Counseling, 4,* 19–31.

Epstein, N. B., Sigal, J. J., & Rakoff, V. (1962). *Family categories schema.* Unpublished manuscript.

Gilligan, J. (1997). *Violence.* New York, NY: Vintage Books.

Grebstein, L. C. (1986). An eclectic family therapy. In J. Norcross (Ed.), *Handbook of eclectic psychotherapy* (pp. 282–319). New York, NY: Brunner/Mazel.

Grossman, H. (1972). *Nine rotten lousy kids.* New York, NY: Holt, Rinehart & Winston.

Guerin, P. J., Jr., & Pendagast, E. G. (1976). Evaluation of family system and genogram. In P. J. Guerin, Jr. (Ed.), *Family therapy: Theory and practice* (pp. 450–464). New York, NY: Gardner Press.

Haley, J. (1972). *Strategies of psychotherapy*. New York, NY: Grune & Stratton.

Haley, J. (1976). *Problem-solving therapy*. San Francisco, CA: Jossey-Bass.

Minuchin, S. (1974). *Families and family therapy*. Cambridge, MA: Harvard University Press.

Minuchin, S., & Fishman, H. C. (1981). *Family therapy techniques*. Cambridge, MA: Harvard University Press.

CHAPTER 8

At the Helm: Interviewing Adolescent Male Juvenile Delinquents

One of the most important tasks of a consultant is interviewing the boys that are referred for a psychological evaluation. Recall from the previous chapters that the overarching philosophy at Ocean Tides is that its residents are perceived as valuable individuals who possess the capacity to overcome the obstacles they have encountered and to learn how to draw upon their own strengths in doing so. An important step in helping them accomplish this is to identify those strengths. Although many of the youngsters have received previous evaluations, either in school or mental health settings, it is important to assess them when they enter the program. They have often encountered new problematic experiences between their most recent evaluation and the time at which they enter the Ocean Tides program.

The decision to include an assessment of referred youngsters as part of the consultant's role was based on two considerations. First, and most important, an individual assessment was considered to be valuable in developing an individualized treatment plan for the resident. Second, when the program first began, no one else on the staff had the necessary clinical experience or advanced training in assessment techniques to do a psychological evaluation. Geffner, Igelman, and Zellner (2003, pp. 5–6) note while referring to patients who have been exposed to parental interpersonal violence that:

> Before treatment is initiated, it is important to make sure an adequate assessment is conducted since all children are not

> the same. It is rare, unfortunately, that programs and shelters actually conduct a comprehensive assessment. Such an assessment should focus on the children's levels of self-esteem, depression, anger, anxiety, trauma, attitudes about power and control, communication and assertiveness skills, and social skills...In order to conduct treatment, the actual issues in need of attention must be known so that the treatment can be tailored to meet the child's varying needs. Further, assessment of the child's strengths and sources of support should also be evaluated in order for areas of resiliency to be identified and built upon in treatment. If we assume one size fits all then our interventions are less likely to be successful or efficient for the particular children we are attempting to help.

Essentially, the boys' individual needs drive the intervention and rehabilitation procedures that are implemented in the Ocean Tides program.

The boys are evaluated within a reasonable time after their arrival, allowing some time to settle in and get used to the new routines. The nature of the evaluation departs from the more formal and traditional mental health interview and is more informal. It became clear in the early stages of working with these young men that they were much less likely to respond to the type of interview used in a mental health setting and required a different approach. Most people seeking help in outpatient mental health or counseling facilities do so voluntarily and are willing to provide information about themselves. The delinquent boys are different. They are often guarded, private, non trusting, suspicious of anything having to do with psychology or psychiatry, and often resentful of being asked about their personal lives.

PHILOSOPHY OF INTERVIEWING

Underlying the approach to interviewing described in this chapter are two fundamental beliefs: One is the importance of individual differences and the other is the importance of identifying a person's strengths in addition to their problems or deficits. The goal is to assess the adolescent's unique personality characteristics that can contribute to helping him change his behavior rather than focus on only assessing psychopathology and reaching a diagnosis. The notion of individual differences, that every person is a unique individual, is one of the foundations of modern psychology. It is this uniqueness among individuals that provides an important and essential ingredient for successful rehabilitation. Being able to identify a young man's unique personality characteristics, and, in particular his strengths, provides a platform on which to build a successful rehabilitative strategy.

This is not as easy as it sounds. By virtue of their backgrounds, including racial and ethnic identity, socioeconomic status, history of behavioral difficulties, family environments, and adjudicated crimes, many delinquents become stereotyped early in their lives and their individual strengths and unique qualities have been forgotten, neglected, or never recognized. If a young man has been evaluated in the past, it is likely that the evaluation emphasizes the negative aspects of his personality and behavior, such as his psychopathology, conflicts, behavior problems, and interpersonal difficulties.

Regardless of how dysfunctional a young man's behavior has been in the past, he has strengths. Often, with adjudicated delinquents, their positive qualities have been minimized or ignored. Although a variety of techniques may be employed in the process of trying to understand the youngster and obtain information, the basic attitude of the interviewer consists of respect and appreciation of the value and uniqueness of the adolescent's life experiences.

THE "CURIOSITY MODEL" OF INTERVIEWING

The style of interviewing delinquents that is described here is called, for lack of a better name, the "curiosity model." Like the young child who mercilessly pursues his or her parent with "why" questions until the curiosity is satisfied, the interviewer asks a variety of specific questions, although rarely "why" questions. It is important to enter the interview with an open mind and a basic attitude of acceptance and respect rather than a preconceived notion of psychopathology or deviant behavior. To achieve this, it is important to not review any information in the youngster's file prior to the interview.

It is a good idea to approach the interview as the legal system approaches a trial—the youngster is considered innocent until he is proven guilty. To clarify, even though the youngster has already been convicted of a crime and his culpability established, the goal is to establish a comfortable atmosphere in which the youngster feels free to tell his story. The initial task is to both engage the youngster and establish a relationship of trust and mutual respect in order to get him to talk openly about himself. When the focus is on identifying and describing weaknesses, deficits, problems, and psychopathology, as it often is in diagnostic or assessment interviews, this can be communicated to the person being interviewed. The result can be that the adolescent either shuts down or responds in kind by revealing only his dark side and problems. Although the assessment of psychopathology has its place and can provide useful and important data, this information is often revealed by prior assessments and reports. This is certainly true with adjudicated delinquents whose histories are often filled with detailed descriptions of their misdeeds that have been documented by teachers, parents, police, probation counselors, and mental health professionals. Conducting a standard psychiatric type of diagnostic interview or mental status interview is a sure way to turn off delinquents and put a quick end to the interview.

KEY ISSUES IN INTERVIEWING DELINQUENTS

Evaluating the personalities and psychological functioning of delinquent adolescents by the use of the interview is a process that is often filled with unexpected and interesting moments. It can be a fairly straightforward procedure that follows the customary path of standard interviewing techniques. When this is the case, no special tips are necessary. However, interviewing delinquent adolescents can be a challenging and difficult task. Consequently, this chapter focuses on the problems and troublesome nature of talking with these youngsters. We provide both rationales and practical strategies for conducting interviews that are useful for rehabilitation plans with court-adjudicated adolescent male juvenile delinquents.

The information in this chapter is based on individual interviews with approximately 1,200 male juvenile delinquents conducted over a period of 40 years. Regardless of the amount of prior experience an interviewer has, it is important to approach each new interview as if it is the first one in order to minimize preconceived notions or biases. It has become almost a cliché of contemporary culture that conversations between adults and teenagers are at best a trying process, and at the worst, a hostile standoff. Although they have different complaints, adults and adolescents seem to agree that it is often hard to have a civil and productive conversation with each other. Teenagers complain that adults are rigid, out of touch with contemporary reality, excessively controlling, or just dumb. Adults complain that teenagers are disrespectful, uncommunicative, sullen, and hostile. The communication gap is often widest between parents and their own children. Although these generalizations do not apply to all adult–adolescent communications, they contain enough truth to foster the belief that both parties *expect* to have trouble talking to each other. This belief often contributes to a self-fulfilling prophecy. Instead of beginning a conversation without bias, both parties often begin with preconceived notions that can prevent a meaningful exchange.

Important Factors in Interviewing Juvenile Delinquents

Lack of Trust of Mental Health Professionals

Juvenile delinquents present a special challenge to the professional mental health interviewer. They tend to be non trusting of anyone outside of their inner circle of friends or family and are particularly wary of "shrinks," which is anyone working in the mental health system regardless of actual professional identity. To put it mildly, these young men are often reluctant to talk to anyone identified as a mental health professional or a counselor. As one youngster succinctly stated with regard to counseling: "I wouldn't go if they sent me and if they forced me to go, I wouldn't say anything." Consequently, delinquents can be guarded, withdrawn, sullen, manipulative, passive-aggressive, openly defiant or hostile, sarcastic, verbally abusive, and noncompliant. In other words, delinquents are not always easy to talk to, and they can try the patience of even the most skilled and experienced interviewer. It is important to point out that delinquents can also be charming, engaging, talkative, and self-disclosing. When this occurs, the interviewer may become suspicious and question the genuineness of the adolescent's behavior. The somewhat cynical belief on the part of the interviewer is that, if the teenager is being pleasant or cooperative, he must have some ulterior motive or is "playing" the interviewer.

The Importance of Noticing Appearance and Behavior in the Interview

The unspoken part of any assessment consists of the interviewer's observation of the interviewee's appearance and behavior during the assessment. It is important to notice and be able to describe the young's man appearance. This includes a description of his physical characteristics, such as his height, body type, and grooming and hair style; how he was dressed; the presence of earrings or other jewelry; any visible piercings or other adornments; and any distinctive marks, such as tattoos, scars, or piercings. Behavior displayed during the interview includes issues such as his cooperation, attitude, mood, and overt behavior. In this sample, we have information about the demeanor of each of the boys' 669 interviews (n = 42.2% of the boys at Ocean Tides). These data reveal that during the consultant's interviews, some of the boys display greater than average unpleasantness, about 15.8% of all the boys at Ocean Tides (n = 250): nervousness (2%, n = 31), seriousness (5.3%, n = 84), intensity (1.3%, n = 20), anxiousness (4.6%, n = 73), sarcasm (0.4%, n = 5), and some are particularly guarded (3.7%, n = 58). Overall, just 5.8% (n = 39) of the boys for whom we have data were uncooperative, 47.7% (n = 319) were moderately cooperative, and 46.5% (n = 311) were very cooperative.

Establishing a Working Relationship

It is the interviewer's task to establish enough of a relationship for a meaningful conversation to take place. This requires not only considerable skills in interviewing, but patience, tact, honesty, ingenuity, creativity and, at times, a good sense of humor. Interviewing juvenile delinquents can be a little like going for a walk in a park or other pleasant environment in which there is a hidden minefield. If you get too comfortable with admiring the surroundings and do not watch your step, the interview can blow up at any time. Keeping your wits about you is essential. Hoge, after reviewing several sources for developing interviewing skills with delinquents, suggests the following general guidelines: establish rapport, listen carefully, remain objective, facilitate communication, maintain control, and avoid argumentation (Hoge, 2008, p. 67). Although these guidelines suggest useful goals for the interview, they do not provide sufficient specific information about how to practically achieve these goals.

TABLE 8.1
How Often a Resident Assumes Responsibility for His Actions

	n	PERCENT OF RESPONDENTS	PERCENT OF ALL OT RESIDENTS
Never	283	17.9	20.6
Sometimes	601	37.9	43.6
Usually	400	25.2	29.0
Always	93	5.9	6.8
Total	1,377	86.9	100
System missing	208	13.1	

OT, Ocean Tides.

By the time youngsters reach the assessment interview, they may have already had a number of negative experiences with other adults, such as parents, teachers, school administrators, police, mental health professionals, and/or other adults in positions of authority. Even though the youngsters have actively contributed to their problems, they often perceive others to be at fault. They may not accept responsibility for their behavior and attribute the blame to external sources, either other persons or the situation. They may genuinely believe that they have been unfairly treated, singled out, discriminated against, and/or victimized by others or "the system." Twenty percent of the Ocean Tides boys overall *never* accept responsibility for their actions (see Table 8.1 for details).

The following anecdote from an interview with an Ocean Tides resident illustrates both a young man's poor impulse control and also his tendency to rationalize or justify his own behavior by externalizing responsibility on to others or the situation.

> We were discussing his participation in a high school wrestling tournament. John said that he would have been All State, but was penalized 40 points for assaulting a referee after he made a call on him that John considered unfair. John said that the referee claimed that his opponent pinned him. John did not like the call and got up and "went after" the referee. He maintained that the referee was a teacher at the same school of his opponent and was therefore biased. John alleged that the videotape of his match supported his claim of unfair officiating.

Regarding this same young man's poor impulse control, he proudly related in the same interview how he had told the principal to "go fuck himself" and walked out of his office after being sent there by a teacher for disruptive behavior in the classroom.

Sometimes a youngster's beliefs are a manipulative ploy to avoid taking responsibility for his behavior. At other times, it may be defensive in the sense that it does not represent a conscious attempt to mislead or deceive others. The interviewer has the difficult task of determining if the youngster's beliefs have a basis in reality or are a distortion. The interviewer may have to maintain a delicate balance between being empathic to the delinquent's complaints and objective enough to sort out the truth.

What the Delinquent Brings to the Interview

One of the first hurdles to overcome in the interview is any negative attitudes or suspicions the youngster has based on prior interactions. As one of the residents stated in referring to a family therapist his family had "forced" him to see: "I didn't like him because he asked a lot of dumb questions." The interviewer responded, "Like me," which got a laugh. Based on their prior interactions with authority figures, which may have been critical or punitive, a resident is likely to have an unfavorable opinion of adults in positions of authority. The adolescent may have experienced a loss of face or felt like he was in a one-down position. This can contribute to the adoption of an adversarial stance characterized by a variety of defensive behaviors, such as overt aggressiveness, passive-aggressiveness, sarcasm, defiance and oppositional behavior, silence, suspiciousness, guardedness, and so on. However, it is interesting to note that in all of the interviews with delinquents that the consultant has conducted, only one young man refused to cooperate to the extent that he walked out of the interview. Ironically, that occurred after the interviewer had complimented him on the hat he was wearing! The young man was returned to the state training school the following week for serious noncompliant behavior in the program.

Textbooks on psychotherapy, particularly psychoanalytically oriented psychotherapy, often warn prospective therapists to be prepared for their clients to attack them personally by identifying some flaw or defect in the therapist in order to throw them off the track when they are getting close to a sensitive issue of the client. Delinquents frequently employ this strategy in an interview. Their behavior can range from open hostility and attacks on the interviewer to noncompliant silence. The delinquent's primary goal is to be self-protective. Self-disclosure is considered to be risky and potentially dangerous. A frequent ploy is to complain, often vehemently, about the unfair and unjust treatment they have received (or continue to receive) from the significant adults in their world. They may be unwilling to accept responsibility for their behavior and attribute the blame for their actions on others. It can be a situation much like a game or a matching of wits in which the interviewer is trying to do everything he or she can think of to get the information and the youngster is trying just as hard to not provide anything meaningful. Simply put, these youngsters can be very difficult to interview. The main task of the interviewer is to find ways to overcome these barriers to communication.

The Interviewer's Attitude: The Importance of Remaining Calm, Patient, and Accepting

Interviewing delinquents can be a trying emotional experience for the interviewer in different ways. It can be very frustrating to try and obtain meaningful information. The delinquents can describe vicious and abhorrent acts of violence with no remorse and even contempt for their victims. As a result, they can stimulate strong feelings of frustration, annoyance, or even anger in an interviewer. It is important that the interviewer recognize these feelings when they arise and not respond by being judgmental or critical. It is imperative that the interviewer resists the temptation to condemn or put down the youngster. At times it takes tremendous discipline and self-restraint to keep from responding in a negative manner. For example, one young man described a robbery in which he and two accomplices assaulted a younger victim to steal a necklace. After knocking the victim to the ground, the young man in the interview, who was wearing heavy work boots at the time of the crime, described how he continued to kick and stomp the other defenseless young man in the head and body to the extent that the victim was later hospitalized with serious injuries. When asked if he had any remorse for his actions, the young man responded that the victim was "stupid" and it was his fault for not voluntarily handing over the jewelry in the first place. Despite the interviewer's personal feelings of revulsion at this senseless, unnecessary, and remorseless act of violence, he had to maintain his professional composure.

These young men can also evoke a very different emotional response from the interviewer; namely, compassion and sadness for the sense of futility and hopelessness they experience. More than one youngster has expressed that he feels doomed because of his environment and the only way to "get out of the life" would be to be able to move to a completely different environment and get a fresh start. This is usually not a realistic option. This is particularly true for the inner city youngsters who are involved in drug trafficking. Many of them have had close friends killed on the street and have also had close encounters with death themselves. Some of the stories that these young men have to tell about their deprived backgrounds and histories of abuse and neglect can be truly heartbreaking. More than one has stated that they do not expect to live past the age of 25 years, if that long.

An example of a particularly sad case occurred a couple of years ago. The consultant had been asked to see one of the residents to determine if it was safe for him to go home for the weekend on his usual pass. A rival gang member had shot a close friend and the resident wanted to visit him in the hospital. The staff was concerned for the resident's safety. In interviewing him, the consultant was impressed by his maturity, commitment to his friend, and determination to visit him. He made it clear that if the staff denied his pass, he would run away from the program. This would have been a shame because he was only a couple of months away from completing the program and being released. He convinced the interviewer that he would be safe. The administrative team allowed him to go home for the weekend and he returned unharmed. Six months after completing the program, he was shot and killed on the street in a revenge shooting by a rival gang. Prior to his untimely death, he had been attending college and staying out of trouble. Another example of a tragic and senseless ending to a life on the mend and filled with promise.

It is important for the interviewer to remain calm, matter-of-fact, candid, and direct. Recognizing that a youngster's adversarial or uncooperative behavior is motivated by a sense of survival or an attempt to achieve self-efficacy can help the interviewer avoid a negative response. A sense of humor can help to diffuse tension and negative interactions. For example, in a recent interview, a youngster convicted of first-degree robbery described how he punched the victim (breaking his nose and cheekbone) and took his iPod because the victim owed him $20. The interviewer asked how taking the iPod was going to get him the money he was owed. The resident said that he was going to return it to the victim after he got the money he was owed. "Sort of like a one man pawn shop," mused the interviewer. They both had a good laugh over the comment and it defused the tension.

As the curiosity model would suggest, curiosity and humility on the part of the interviewer are qualities that can help facilitate a productive interview. Regardless of the number of assessments an interviewer may have conducted, talking with these young men is rarely dull, uninteresting, or routine. They often reveal talents and skills that are surprising and deserving of admiration or at least respect, even though they may be used for ill-begotten purposes. In dealing with the frustration of a particularly nonresponsive youngster, the interviewer must at times accept the fact that the interview is not going anywhere. No matter how skilled or experienced the interviewer, there are times when an interviewer is going to strike out with a particular young man. On those occasions when the interviewer might feel especially frustrated by being outwitted, outmaneuvered, or blocked by a youngster, it is important to have some inner resource for remaining calm and in good humor. Sometimes, things just do not go as well as intended and the best thing to do is to preserve enough of the relationship to try again another day. In a residential program, that opportunity will arise again.

Conducting the Interview

The Referral Process

Before describing the actual conduct of an interview, it is helpful to describe the context in which the interview occurs. The director of social services gives the consultant a list of recently arrived residents and the consultant interviews the youngsters in the order on the list. Sometimes the order is changed when the teachers or other staff members feel that a certain youngster should have priority because of adjustment difficulties in the program. If a resident has made suicidal threats or has given other indications of potentially harming himself or others, this is an immediate reason for referral, even for a resident who has already been interviewed.

The Introduction Phase

Usually, the consultant goes to the classroom and takes the resident to the interview room. After introducing himself, the consultant asks the youngster if the youngster has seen him before. Sometimes, the young man's response provides a prediction of how the interview will go. As the consultant usually interviews the residents several weeks to several months after they have entered the program, they have had the opportunity to see the consultant on the premises. When a resident indicates that he has seen the consultant around, it is often a sign that he will be more cooperative and talkative once the interview begins. This is not always the case. Some residents say that they have seen the consultant, but have no idea of who the consultant is or what the consultant does. Regardless of the response, the interviewer tells the resident that he is a consultant and explains that a consultant is a person who comes in from the outside to work with the staff. The consultant tells the resident that he is at Ocean Tides every Friday morning to meet with the teachers and other staff. The purpose of the interview is for the consultant to get to know the resident so that the consultant will be more informed if the young man is discussed at one of the staff meetings the consultant attends. Specifically, the consultant often says that he wants the resident to be more than "a name on a piece of paper." The interviewer indicates that he will be asking the resident lots of questions and emphasizes that this will probably be the only time that they will talk individually.

The fact that this is their only contact is often reassuring to the youngsters because it is well known among the residents that the consultant is in reality "the shrink." Although some newly arrived residents say that they do not know the professional identity of the consultant, they quickly find out through the grapevine. For example, when the consultant goes to a class and requests to see a youngster, one of the other residents will sometimes yell out: "Oh, you're going to see the shrink." It is interesting that rarely does a resident ask the consultant if he is "a shrink" or question the consultant about his professional identity. If a young man asks the consultant if he is a psychologist or psychiatrist, the consultant tells the resident. It is interesting to note that the consultant can count on the fingers of one hand the number of residents who have ever asked about his professional identity.

The reason the consultant does not tell youngsters that he is a psychologist is because that is almost a guarantee of their lack of cooperation or silence. As previously noted, most of the delinquents are contemptuous of the mental health system and its representatives. Many have experienced prior outpatient counseling, brief hospitalizations in psychiatric hospitals, and/or mental health evaluations. They almost always have negative comments about these experiences. Although in many cases their reactions are clearly defensive and self-protective, the simple fact is that they do not like to talk to anyone they consider to be associated with the mental health system. These kids often adhere to a "macho" code of silence. If they perceive the interview as an attempt to get them to provide any meaningful information about themselves, their families, or their friends, they clam up and do not say anything.

Regardless of the interviewer's comments, many youngsters approach the interview with skepticism, distrust, and an oppositional stance. In order to counter this attitude, the consultant approaches the youngster with deference, respect, and in a down-to-earth, matter-of-fact manner. A facade of bravado, nonchalance, arrogance, or disdain on a youngster's part may mask underlying feelings of incompetence, insecurity, and uncertainty. It is important to recognize this and not to treat the youngster in any way that he might consider as being "put down." On the contrary, to conduct a successful interview, it is important to help the youngster to feel accepted, confident, secure, and in control. This is particularly important at the outset. Getting off on the right foot is critical. The beginning of the interview often creates the tone that will determine the remainder of the conversation.

Beginning the Interview

In order to create a neutral and nonthreatening context for the interview, the interviewer begins by telling the resident that he knows nothing about the resident, which is the truth. The interviewer follows this opening with simple factual questions, such as: "How long have you been in the program?" or "Did you come from home or the training school?" It is important to begin with factual types of questions that the youngster can answer easily. These opening questions are followed with questions about the boy's home life and family, such as: "Where do you live?" and "Who's at home?" By asking simple and nonthreatening questions that can be easily answered, the interviewer gives the young man an opportunity to demonstrate his competence. In addition, the interviewer is trying to communicate a message at the meta-communication level.

Namely, the purpose of the interview is not to embarrass, intimidate, or harass the young man, but to give him the opportunity to demonstrate his knowledge, competence, and worth as a person. In the beginning, the questions are very specific. For example, if the young man responds vaguely to a question about his home by naming a city, the interviewer will ask the resident more specifically to describe his neighborhood or street. As a native of and long-term resident of the state, the consultant will use his familiarity with the resident's neighborhood to have a brief conversation about where the boy lives. Obviously, if the interviewer is unfamiliar with the location of the boy's home, this approach is not viable and an alternative strategy is to ask the young man to describe his home environment in more detail. The consultant probably spends more time talking about these specifics than many interviewers might, but his purpose is to try and ground the person, both literally and figuratively. By discussing familiar landmarks and other details of the resident's home environment, the consultant has a better chance of moving from the position of a distant authority figure to within a more personal, and hopefully acceptable, place.

Engaging the Adolescent

In outpatient psychotherapy engaging the client was the most important, but often neglected, aspect of successful psychotherapy. Research has shown that a significant percent of clients who voluntarily sought outpatient psychotherapy did not return for a second visit. Similarly, getting off on the right foot is a key ingredient in a successful interview with a juvenile delinquent. This involves finding a way to engage the youngster in a process he is suspicious of and one in which he is reluctant to participate. It is important to find a topic early in the interview that the young man is willing to discuss. This may be an area of interest or a source of pride, even if it involves an aspect of negative behavior, such as providing details about his crimes, his drug use, or other exploits.

The young man's appearance can provide clues for fruitful areas to explore. Simple observations, such as a comment about how the young man is dressed, can be a potential icebreaker. Adolescents often use their physical appearance as a way to attract attention or to express their individuality. Youngsters who call attention to their appearance in some obvious way may want to be noticed and are often willing to talk at length about this. Unusual hairstyles, carefully trimmed beards or other special grooming, facial or body piercing, earrings or other jewelry, and visible tattoos provide effective conversations starters. About 6% (*n* = 99) of the residents that the consultant has interviewed at Ocean Tides had visible piercings and 4% (*n* = 64) had visible tattoos. For example, a 17-year-old African American resident, who described his racial identity as "regular Black," had the letters "R. I. P." tattooed on the back of his hand. He explained that it stood for his uncle, who was shot when he was 24 years old. The same young man had a tattoo on his other forearm of a pair of praying hands with the name "Chris" beneath them. This tattoo was in memory of his younger brother who died in an automobile accident when he was 10 years old.

Many of these boys have experienced considerable loss. Our data identify 35.3% (*n* = 560) of the Ocean Tides boys as having already experienced the death of someone significant in their lives. Sometimes, the tattoos are self-explanatory as in the case of the resident who had the letters "thug" on the upper backs of the fingers of his left hand and the word "life" on the fingers of his right hand. The term "thug" is from the hip hop community and was coined by the late rap artist Tupac Shakur. Shakur's acronym for "Thug Life" is The Hate U Give Lil' Infants F**ks Everybody. Following Shakur's death, Thug Life became a movement. "Thug Life" became a phrase meaning "the life one must lead in order to rise through the everyday struggle." It refers to anyone who attempts to arise from poverty, adversity, or despair.

Another resident had a cross with the name "Joey D." under it on his upper arm. This tattoo commemorated the memory of his best friend who had been killed in a motorcycle accident. Another tattoo was of a pair of wings on the back of a resident's neck. When the interviewer commented on that, the resident rolled up the sleeves of his jersey and revealed tattoos on both arms that extended from just above the wrists to his shoulders. On his left arm he had the four Chinese symbols for knowledge, eternity, wisdom, and trust, and another large tattoo above these with his name in the middle. On his right arm, he had a tattoo with his late grandfather's name and a series of other tattoos running down his arm, including the words "love and hate" on his forearm.

It is important that any comments made by the interviewer be sincere and not offered in a manner that might be interpreted as patronizing, sarcastic, or condescending. Remarks do not have to be positive or complimentary. Neutral comments, such as "That's an interesting tattoo you have, tell me about it" can be effective. Regardless of their overt responses, adolescents are often pleased to have their appearance noticed. This can be an effective way to open a conversation and establish rapport or to explore a personally meaningful experience that might not otherwise be apparent. When an interviewer acknowledges the manner in which a youngster is presenting himself, it is an affirmation of the adolescent's values and identity. Regardless of what they may admit, many adolescents are very sensitive about what others think of them. If they suspect the interviewer is insincere or merely using a technique, they will respond negatively in some way.

Creating a Window of Opportunity

"Creating a window of opportunity" is an extension of the engagement techniques just described and involves finding a topic the delinquent is willing to talk about in detail or more openly. This may be an interest or an area of competence that, ironically, might involve his criminal offenses. Delinquents often take pride in elaborating about their misdeeds and exploits. It is one of the few topics that they might discuss in detail and reveal information voluntarily and spontaneously. If a young man is resistant to answering factual questions about his family, which happens occasionally but is unusual, asking about existing charges is often a good way to begin for several reasons. Their charges are a matter of public record and a reason for their being in custody so that they know this is information that is available to staff. They do not feel as if they are providing any new information. Asking about offenses gets right to the point and communicates the interviewer's directness and willingness to deal with relevant issues. Discussion of charges also offers the youngster the opportunity to tell his side of the story. In some cases, they are embarrassed, remorseful, or ashamed of their behavior. The down side to this approach is that you have to take what they tell you with a grain of salt because their reports are often prone to distortion. This can include exaggerating or even making up stories for shock value, or at the other extreme and more commonly, denying or minimizing the nature of the offenses. It is interesting to note that not all youngsters are willing to describe or discuss their charges in any detail.

The young man's perceptions of his own behavior are inseparable from the reactions to it by others, as explained by labeling theory in criminology. He internalizes the deviant label and thus attempts to live up to expectations in society for what it means to be deviant or criminal. Adopting the deviant identity gives him purpose, a sense of self that is reinforced by the shocked reactions of others when he tells his stories or recounts his deeds, no matter how truthful they are. By talking about their charges, though, they can simultaneously emphasize their competencies and communicate their disdain for conventional society and its rules.

Listening carefully and asking leading questions, regardless of the content of the information being discussed, can provide useful information. This is one of the times in the interview when it is important for the interviewer to carefully monitor his or her own emotional reactions and inhibit communicating any personal feelings of judgment or disapproval. One of the few certainties in dealing with delinquents is that they have already experienced prior negative judgments, criticism, disapproval, or punishment for their behavior and/or attitudes. One of the fastest ways to turn a delinquent off and shut down the interview is to react negatively to what he is telling you. This does not mean that humor or benign skepticism cannot be used. As an interviewer gains experience in dealing with delinquents, he or she establishes internal norms or parameters for behavior that can serve as useful guidelines to evaluate the credibility of what is being said. So when a young man says something highly unlikely, such as he smokes an ounce of pot a day by himself, a skeptical "really?" or similar challenge can be an effective and appropriate response. This can be followed by a request for more details on how the young man finds the time to smoke that much, where he gets the money to afford that amount of marijuana, and similar questions.

Discussing the details of offenses provides an opportunity to assess the talents and skills of the delinquent that might not be apparent in other ways. School grades and other more conventional measures of achievement, including psychological testing, are often inaccurate indications of a youngster's talents and abilities because of lack of motivation and effort. A more accurate measure of youngsters' true talents may be provided by the skills they employ in their criminal activities. When discussing this topic, curiosity is often the best guide for questioning. As most interviewers do not come from criminal backgrounds, they know little about the actual procedures employed in committing crimes, except for what they may have learned from reading or talking to offenders. Asking about this can empower the young man by making him the expert and provide valuable insight about his talents and abilities that are not otherwise evident. Asking specific questions about techniques, strategies, motivations, and results of the youngster's crimes can provide valuable insights. The interviewer's experience is that the young men respond positively to detailed questions more often than not. A fringe benefit of this approach is that sometimes the interviewer can acquire information that is practically useful. For example, one consultant once locked his keys in his car after a quick stop at a supermarket on his way to his private office. He was able to open the car door without any damage to the vehicle by utilizing a rather simple technique that an accomplished car thief had once described to him. Any topic that suggests an area of a delinquent's interests or source of pride is a potentially fruitful subject for facilitating a productive interview.

Playing Dumb: A Useful Technique

A late friend and colleague, who was a wonderfully perceptive and effective clinical psychologist, had a favorite saying: "Everyone is dumb about something every day." Translated: Regardless of how much we know, at any given moment, we can all fail to remember something important or to ask a particular question. Sometimes, the interview takes on the quality of a game. This can take the form of playful humor, such as the convicted thief who, observing a marble-top corner table with a nice lamp on it in the interview room, commented: "That would really look nice in my room. I think I'll take it back with me." Some adolescents, particularly intelligent ones, approach the interview as a challenge to outwit or mislead the interviewer. The following vignette illustrates this point.

> The interviewee was an extremely bright 17-year old African American young man. Prior psychological testing indicated a full scale Wechsler IQ in the 130s. He came from a good home with two loving, highly successful parents. Both his mother and father had attained very high administrative positions in a public school system. Despite this apparently supportive background and his natural talent, he had a long history of self-defeating behavior and participation in crime. During the interview, the consultant asked him about his career plans. He responded that he wanted to be "an assassin." The interviewer

> responded with curiosity about his choice, explaining that he could understand wanting to be a "hit man," because there was good money in it. He added that this young man was the first resident who had ever told him he wanted to be an assassin and they discussed this for a brief spell. The young man was clearly taken aback by his failure to either shock or get a rise out of the interviewer. After the interview, one of the residential staff overheard the delinquent commenting to his peers about the interview: "Who was that guy?" he said. "I tried to fuck with his head and he fucked with mine!" It is interesting to note that this young man, after successfully completing the program, was re-arrested for a minor crime the night before his scheduled induction into the Marine Corps.

A frequently used approach to interviewing that is useful with delinquent adolescents is a variation of Socratic questioning called the "Columbo Technique." The name comes from the TV series of the 1970s in which Peter Falk played Lieutenant Columbo, a detective who intentionally masked his astute sleuthing skills with a bumbling facade. Sobell and Sobell (2008) describe the technique as follows. "The Columboesque approach is intended as a curious inquiry about discrepant behaviors without being judgmental or blaming and allows for the juxtaposing in a nonconfrontational manner of information that is contradictory." In other words, this is a type of "playing dumb" in which the interviewer asks questions in a self-derisive manner while apologizing for his or her ignorance and ineptitude. This is an easy approach for a professional consultant to use with delinquents because the consultant may in fact be exploring topics about which he or she knows very little.

Another useful tactic is the use of benign skepticism indicated by a raised eyebrow, questionable glance, or skeptical comment, such as "Really?" This is particularly useful in dealing with suspected manipulators or con artists or in challenging exaggerated reports of drug use. Finally, admitting to actual ignorance by acknowledging to the youngster that he does not in fact know or understand something can be very helpful. When an interviewer admits ignorance about a particular subject candidly, the youngster being interviewed will often respond with a detailed explanation. For example, a young man being interviewed insisted that he was not in a gang despite the interviewer's beliefs to the contrary. The interviewer said something to the effect that, having never been in a gang, he did not know much about how they operated. He asked the young man if they were run like businesses that had a boss who ran things and gave orders to the workers. The young man immediately responded with a detailed mini-lecture on how most gangs were organized and run, but that the gang he belonged to was different. He then explained in detail how his gang operated.

This technique also has the effect of genuinely empowering the interviewee so that he does not feel in a "one-down" position. This enhances the relationship and can facilitate a more productive interview. However, this approach is not always successful. Because of their low self-esteem, many youngsters find it hard to "accept being accepted." For example, after the consultant told one young man that he found him to be "interesting," the resident responded: "Do you say that to everybody?"

Content Areas for the Interview

Although the order in which an interviewer discusses topics varies with the individual, there are certain areas that are routinely explored in an assessment interview. These include family composition and history, including where the family lives; current charges and prior offenses, including the youngster's emotional responses to his crimes (e.g., any feelings of guilt or remorse); drug and alcohol use; school experiences and work history; career goals and plans; recreational interests and hobbies, including participation in organized sports or other activities, activities with peers, and romantic/sexual interests and experiences; prior placements, counseling and/or mental health treatment, including previous hospitalizations and medications; a brief mental status screening, particularly for depression. The latter topic always includes questions about prior, recent, or current suicidal attempts or ideation. Additional topics may include sexual history and experiences: any history of sexual, emotional, or physical abuse or neglect; significant losses; religious and spiritual orientation; and any unique or idiosyncratic experiences of significance in the young man's life. As there is likely to be information on these topics available in the youngster's medical, school, and legal records, the main purpose of the interview is to ascertain the young man's perspective and to form impressions based on his responses.

One of the best indications of a youngster's sincerity and truthfulness is the extent to which the information he provides in the interview is consistent with the information in his file. Following an interview with the youngster, the consultant writes a formal report that includes the reason for the referral; a detailed description of his behavior during the interview (behavioral observations), a summary of these content areas organized under separate headings (family; charges; substance use; interests, plans for the future, and prior school adjustment; prior treatment; impressions); a diagnosis using the latest *Diagnostic and Statistical Manual of Mental Disorders* classification; and a section on recommendations. Following are some comments describing how the consultant approaches each content area.

Family

This is usually the first topic and is a crucial area because many of the youngsters come from complicated, chaotic, and dysfunctional families, or, as Kagan and Schlosberg (1989) labeled them, "Families in Perpetual Crisis." When this is the case, they are often reluctant to talk in detail about their families because they are embarrassed. It is necessary to proceed with caution and tact. The consultant almost always begins by asking where the youngster lives. Depending on the boy's response, he may ask more specific questions about the particular neighborhood, if it is in one of the larger cities. Following this, he asks who is at home and the ethnic–racial identity of the youngster and his parents. Many of the delinquents come from mixed ethnic and racial backgrounds. It is important to see if the youngster knows this information and is willing to provide it. In discussing the youngster's family, the interviewer tries to obtain simple, nonthreatening factual information. This includes the questions about the parents and their work, ages, and activities (i.e., school or occupations) of siblings in the home or out of the home, including all step- and half-siblings. If it is a single-parent family, the interviewer inquires if the parent is divorced, widowed, or never married. If the young man was born out of wedlock, which is more often the norm than the exception, the interviewer asks if the young man knows the identity of the missing biological parent, if he has any contact with that parent, and his emotional reaction to the missing parent. Responses to this last question range from avoidance ("I don't know") to indifference or anger.

Many delinquents have experienced significant parental losses as a result of abandonment, death, divorce, incarceration in prison, drug abuse, incapacity due to physical or mental illness, or neglect. This is a difficult but important topic to explore and youngsters will talk about this with varying degrees of openness. In some cases of parental absence or incompetence, the young man has taken on the role of a parental child and has the responsibility of providing care for younger siblings or contributing to the family's income. One of the attractions of and stated motivations for drug dealing is that it provides a lucrative source of income to help the family finances.

Contrary to popular stereotype, not all delinquents come from dysfunctional families. Some come from intact and reasonably stable homes in which there are well-intentioned parents who may have been rendered ineffective by the delinquent's behavior. It is not unusual for delinquents to blame others, particularly parents, for their behavior. Occasionally, a youngster will accept responsibility for his behavior. For example, one young man clearly stated that, although his parents were divorced and remarried to different spouses, they had tried everything they could to help him. With obvious pride he stated that they had filed a total of 32 wayward petitions in attempting to exert some control over his behavior.

Trying to find out about family conflicts and disagreements can be a trying task. Some youngsters will talk openly about their anger or disdain for a parent or stepparent, but others will handle the topic with avoidance and denial. When delinquents do talk about conflicts with parental figures, the youngsters often attribute the blame for the problems to the parent. The most frequent complaints are that the parent is excessively controlling or unreasonable in his or her expectations. Often, delinquents experience normal limit setting and appropriate discipline as unacceptable. This is especially true when initiated by a stepparent.

Responses to questions about their parents can vary enormously. Some young men are very protective of their parents and are reluctant to describe them in a negative light, even when this would be accurate. For example, one young man described his father as an alcoholic, but emphasized that he was able to function. As evidence of this, he said: "He can hold the steering wheel of a car steady and drive fine even after drinking 20 beers." A youngster that had experienced considerable physical abuse by his father on a continuing basis made excuses for his father by stating: "He's a good dad, he just makes bad decisions." Another young man with a seriously mentally ill mother indicated that his mother was "a little crazy." When asked what he meant, he said: "Let's put it this way—she acts as if she has a head full of helium." He meant by this that she was kind of spacey. Despite the fact that his mother had repeated hallucinations, delusions, and had been diagnosed as schizophrenic, he denied that she had a serious mental problem and was only "nervous." A 16-year-old Latino youngster dismissed his father's chronic drinking, infidelity, and recent beating up of his wife by indicating that both his parents worked long hours and had given him "a good life." A young man, whose mother was being treated for anxiety and depression and was on six different psychotropic medications, admitted that his mother had auditory hallucinations and believed that there were people hiding under her bed. He had not mentioned these psychotic symptoms to his mother's psychiatrist and asked the interviewer if these symptoms were side effects of the medications she was taking. Other youngsters express mixed feelings, like the young man who said of his father: "He's an asshole, but I love him."

Youngsters are not always kind or protective of their parents. Sometimes, they go to the other extreme. One young man who came from an upper-middle-class home and whose father was a successful businessman expressed considerable resentment toward his father. Specifically, he felt that his father had too high and unrealistic expectations for him. He described his father as "one of a kind" who was demanding, condescending, insulting, rigid, stubborn, and strong willed.

Relationships with siblings and with the extended family are often significant and should be explored. Sometimes this information will come up spontaneously. For example, one young man was describing his anger at his mother for being unreasonably rigid in her attempts to control him. In the context of this discussion, he mentioned that he had a younger stepsister that he was concerned about because she was "completely under the wing of my mother." His concern was that his sister was so overprotected that "she's not going to be able to handle the real world when she gets older." This description provided valuable insight into this young man's capacity for concern and empathy for others and provided a basis for future counseling. Sometimes, a youngster will mention being close with a grandparent, aunt, uncle, or an adult outside the family who functions as a significant parental figure. These relationships should be explored. If the youngster does not spontaneously mention any such relationship, the interviewer should ask if there is any particular adult with whom the adolescent is close.

Charges

This is one of the easiest topics to inquire about because it is a matter of recorded fact. How the delinquent talks about his charges often provides a barometer for how the rest of the interview will proceed. For example, if the young man is excessively guarded, which is usually indicated by comments such as "I don't know, I can't remember," or "It's in my file," this is a pretty good indication that he will not be forthcoming or truthful about other topics. In addition to being vague, delinquents often minimize the seriousness or extent of their offenses. "Peeling the onion" or asking specific and detailed questions is necessary to obtain a clear picture of what actually happened.

In asking about charges, it is also important to ask about the delinquent's sentence. Sometimes, there is a big discrepancy between the reported charge and the sentence. When this occurs, a follow-up comment or question about this discrepancy can reveal significant new information, such as prior charges. Similarly, vague or general responses should be followed up with questions. Violations of probation charges always indicate prior difficulties. When there is a pattern of criminal behavior, it is important to ask how old the young man was when he first started getting into trouble. A frequent response to this question is some variation of "with the law" or otherwise? The interviewer should ask for both. Another question that is useful to ask, particularly when the delinquent behavior was of sudden onset or represented a significant change from previous behavior, is: "What happened that you suddenly started getting into trouble?" or "How did you go from an honor student to going to jail?"

Asking delinquents how they happen to have been caught or apprehended almost always yields useful and interesting information. Their responses to this question can provide valuable insight into their judgment, problem-solving abilities, level of impulsivity, willingness to accept responsibility for their behavior, and their peer relationships. For example, in a recent interview, a young man reported that he and an accomplice had beaten and robbed a victim. He was arrested as he and his friend were walking down the street and a police car drove by. "Why did the police stop and want to talk to you?" asked the consultant. "I was wearing a red bandanna around my neck," he answered "and the guy we beat up told the police that one of them was wearing a red bandanna. If I had taken the bandanna off, I wouldn't have been caught."

Two related areas to a young man's offenses that are important to explore are his feelings about his crimes and his ownership of his actions. Contrary to popular perceptions, most delinquents are raised by parents who do not want them to commit crimes. They attend schools and are socialized to believe that they should follow rules in society. So before a crime is committed, certain rationalizations occur. Sykes and Matza (1957) explain that anticipated guilt is neutralized to enable deviant behavior, and these techniques are learned. They include denial of responsibility, injury, and/or a victim, condemnation of the condemners, and appeal to higher loyalties. For example, in cases of assault associated with robbery, the perpetrator may indicate that the victim did not voluntarily give up the money or object to being robbed, so the victim "deserved" or asked for the assault; an example of denial of a victim. Does the delinquent accept responsibility or put the blame on others or blame the situation? In asking about this, it is important to remember that this is a diagnostic and not a therapeutic interview. If the young man does not acknowledge responsibility or any remorse, the purpose of the interview is not to pursue this with the goal of changing his attitude, but to find out how he is feeling about it at the current moment. Retaliation against "snitches" is often rationalized in this way. In some cases, the young men claim that the only reason they were apprehended was because someone "snitched." Their idea of "snitching" can involve considerable distortion of reality at times. For example, one young man, who threatened his girlfriend and physically assaulted her friend, considered their reporting his behavior to the police as "snitching." He had no remorse for his actions and expected them to tolerate his violence. He interpreted their going to the police as a personal betrayal.

It is important to verify an adolescent's description of his charges. Although most delinquents that the consultant has interviewed describe their charges in reasonably accurate terms, sometimes they minimize and sometimes they exaggerate. A young man who initially said he was in custody for a "weapons charge" provides a good example of exaggeration. He explained that he had shot someone in his neighborhood with a shotgun. When asked if the victim was seriously injured, he initially responded that he did not know but quickly added that he probably killed the victim because he had used "solid slugs" rather than pellets as ammunition. His motivation for shooting the victim was that "he was a crack addict who owed me money for some cocaine I sold him." His police record indicated only charges of larceny and possession of a firearm. This same young man provided further evidence of exaggeration by stating that he was a highly successful drug dealer who earned $5,000 a week. He maintained that he sold heroin, marijuana, powder cocaine, and crack cocaine, but had never been apprehended or charged for drug dealing. When asked what he did with all the money he earned, he stated that he bought houses and cars. At different times he had owned a Chevy SS and a Mercedes, and currently owned a Cadillac Escalade. When asked what his parents thought about his having such an expensive car, he said they did not know about it because he kept it on an adjacent lot. Another 16-year-old alleged drug dealer, who claimed to "specialize" in selling Ecstasy, estimated that he sold as many as 1,000 pills a week. He claimed to earn between $7,000 and $10,000 a week and used the money to support his girlfriend by paying for her apartment, car, food, and other expenses.

Drug Use

Alcohol and marijuana are the overwhelming choices of drugs by the Ocean Tides boys prior to getting into legal trouble. Although many teenagers use these substances in moderation or on a "recreational" basis, delinquents are much more likely to use them to excess. The use of other drugs, such as amphetamines, Ecstasy, barbiturates, and hallucinogens, occurs less frequently and is usually associated with young men who have a primary substance abuse problem. Surprisingly, relatively few of the delinquents interviewed at Ocean Tides have admitted to using either cocaine or heroin, even on a trial or experimental basis.

The use of drugs is associated with delinquency in several ways. It may be the source of their offenses. That is, the young man may have been charged with either possession of an illegal drug or possession with intent to deliver. Drugs can provide a motive for committing a crime to the extent that the young man needs money to purchase drugs. In the criminological literature, this is called an economic compulsive crime (Salekin & Alexander, 1991). The delinquent may have been under the influence of drugs when he committed the crime or was apprehended. The poor judgment or poor planning involved might have resulted from drug use (known as a "psychopharmacological" drug crime). The use of drugs can interfere with the development of competencies in more socially accepted pursuits, such as performance in school, athletics, or work. Some youngsters use drugs to self-medicate psychological problems like anxiety, depression, and hyperactivity. Finally, a significant number of drug-related crimes are systemic, meaning they arise through the context of competition among drug users and the unregulated nature of the market.

Discussing drug use with delinquents is tricky because they can be so variable in their responses. It can be hard to get an accurate picture. Responses to questions about drug use range from total denial to what appears to be gross exaggerations or flaunting. Following are some illustrations of likely inflated reports of drug use.

> Eddy stated that he smokes between one-half to one ounce of marijuana every day with a couple of his friends. He described in detail and with an air of personal accomplishment how he would smoke before school, during school, and after school. Eddy said he was stoned all day every day. He said that he did not have to buy marijuana because he has a lot of "rich friends" who supplied him.
>
> Kevin admitted that he used to be a heavy user of marijuana and used to spend $400 a week on pot. When he got up in the morning, he would roll 20 Dutch Master blunts and keep them in a cigarette pack. He reported that he had two packs: one contained actual cigarettes and the other contained marijuana blunts. Basically, he was stoned all the time.
>
> David admitted to daily use of marijuana. He said that he would smoke "bowls of good stuff," which he defined as hydroponically grown.
>
> To say that Benny is a heavy user of marijuana would not do him justice. Using marijuana is the single most important activity in his life and is the core of his existence. Benny reported that he initially began using marijuana when he was 9 or 10 years old and has been using it heavily on a daily basis since that time. He cannot remember how he got started. He uses so much that he could not even estimate how much he smokes on a daily basis. As an example, he said that he and his friend purchased about 25 lbs last summer. They sold half, but smoked the rest of it in 3 months. Even if he was

> exaggerating the exact amount of his use, there is no question that it is extensive. When asked what he liked about using pot, he said "everything" and went on to describe the cleaning process, pulling apart the tangles, the preparation, the rolling of joints, etc. He agreed that the use of marijuana is a "style of life" for him.
>
> It was difficult to obtain specific information about the amount and frequency of Toby's drug usage because he said that he could not remember the details. He stated that he smoked "a lot" of pot and started when he was 15. He said that he no longer smokes. At first he said that he smoked "15 blunts a day," but reduced his claim to "10 blunts a day" after the interviewer commented that his report sounded excessive. In a prior evaluation, he admitted to smoking 2 or 3 blunts a day. Toby does not know for how long he smoked. He said the pot relaxed him, but he was "a rowdy drunk."
>
> Quincy indicated that he started smoking marijuana at age 11 and admitted to being a regular and heavy user—about nine blunts a day. He stated: "You're going to think I am exaggerating but I was smoking between a quarter- and a half-ounce every day." He admitted to doing a little selling, but said that he was able to pay for the pot with the money he made from his part-time employment. He discontinued his use of marijuana when his pregnant girlfriend gave him an ultimatum about not smoking if he was going to be a decent father.
>
> Mike estimated that he smoked "between one-quarter and one-half" ounce of marijuana daily as well as frequently drinking strong alcohol, such as "Everclear" (grain alcohol). He reported that the most he ever smoked was "28 blunts" (approximately an ounce of marijuana) in 1 hour with four of his friends.

What is common is that youngsters rarely admit that they may have a problem with drugs even when they acknowledge in detail that they use a particular drug frequently and in large amounts. For example, in talking with a high school athlete of considerable proficiency who admitted to heavy daily use of marijuana, the interviewer asked him if the pot interfered with his ability to play sports. On the contrary, the young man maintained that he played better because he was less nervous and the pot calmed him. In assessing drug use, it is important that the interviewer not only have good interviewing technique, but also a solid knowledge about the effects of drug use itself. This is essential in order to make an accurate assessment about possible drug abuse or dependency.

Asking directly and specifically about drug use frequently will not yield good results. A better strategy is to wait for an opening provided by discussions of other topics or for a suggestive comment by the youngster. For instance, when discussing charges, if the situation sounds like poor judgment or impulsive behavior was involved, the interviewer can ask the young man if he was high at the time. Sometimes a delinquent will volunteer that information even without being asked. He may casually mention in passing that he and his friends were "high," "stoned," or "drunk" at the time of the crime.

In talking about interests and hobbies, a frequent comment is: "I like to hang out with my friends." Asking what they do when they hang out or if they ever get high together is a natural way to broach the topic. If a young man refers to "partying" with his friends, this is an invitation to ask about the nature of the partying. In asking about drugs, it is important to try and maintain a matter-of-fact and almost nonchalant attitude. For example, a simple question like asking a youngster what he likes to drink will yield an interesting response. Most youngsters answer this question by referring to the brand name of a particular drink rather than the type of beverage. This question was initially asked almost as an afterthought by the consultant many years ago. To his surprise, the young man being interviewed reported he liked to drink "Hennessey." Since then, the consultant has found this is a favorite beverage among the delinquents he has interviewed even though most of them do not even know that it is a brand of cognac. They drink it or say they drink it because of the prestige associated with the brand. "Hennessey" is the "Jordan's" of alcohol. In discussing alcohol use, the consultant first tries to determine if the young man drinks at all, and, if so, how much and how often. If the consultant suspects drinking may be an issue, he asks if the youngster has ever "gotten sick," passed out, or been taken to the emergency department.

Some youngsters completely deny any use of alcohol, marijuana, or any other drugs. When this occurs, a useful response can be: "You've never tried pot?" or "You've never had anything to drink?" Usually, the discussion that follows provides a context for interpreting the accuracy and truthfulness of the young man's claim. Having said that, it is important to realize that this is a subject that youngsters often lie about and do so in a convincing manner. Ironically, some of the biggest fabrications involved descriptions of excessive use that stretch credibility, like when a young man reports that he smokes an ounce of marijuana by himself every day. One ounce of marijuana makes approximately 60 cigarettes. That would equate to smoking almost four marijuana cigarettes an hour every waking hour of every day.

Prior School Experiences

Most delinquents have a history of not doing well in school either academically or behaviorally. Previous research (West & Farrington, 1973) indicates that teachers' ratings of troublesome behavior in school are the best single predictors of juvenile delinquency. Typically, delinquents are extremely negative and hostile in their descriptions of past school experiences. They attribute much of the blame for their difficulties to external causes, such as teachers, administrators, or "the system." In asking youngsters about their school experiences, it is important to initially "hear them out" about their complaints in order to try and defuse some of their anger. It is also important to avoid stereotyping about a youngster's attitudes toward school or his or her abilities. For example, in walking with one resident on their way to the interview room, the interviewer noticed that he was carrying a copy of Aldous Huxley's *Brave New World*. The consultant asked if he had ever read George Orwell's book *1984* (the young man had). The interviewer commented that Orwell wrote another interesting book and the delinquent responded "*Animal Farm*." The interviewer commented that he was thinking of an autobiographical description of Orwell's life as a hobo during the Depression. The delinquent responded with the correct name of the book (*Down and Out in Paris and London*) and said that he had read it. When the interviewer commented that the adolescent seemed to be well read, he said, "Not really." Although this incident is not typical, it served as an important reminder not to make negative assumptions about a young man's orientation toward learning.

Asking benign factual questions about where the boy went to school prior to entering the program, what grade he was in, and if that is the appropriate grade is a useful way to begin talking about school experiences. Most youngsters will reveal if they have repeated a grade and what grades they have repeated. The next task is to find out why the young man repeated a grade. To get an answer to this question, the interviewer may have to provide several options, such as: Did you not do the work, not go to school, or try to do the work and found it too difficult. By the time they come to Ocean Tides, many young men have already developed a negative self-fulfilling prophecy about their school performance and have given up on it. They may have feelings of futility or hopelessness and have given up trying to pass in school. The consultant always asks if the young man wants to finish high school and, if not, what he plans to do in the future. The responses here are extremely variable from wanting to graduate high school and go on to college, to obtaining a high school equivalency diploma or to dropping out and going to work. It is not unusual for a young man to say that school is useless.

There are a variety of reasons why delinquents do poorly in school. One of the main reasons is low self-esteem or a failure to believe that they can be successful even when there is compelling evidence that they have the ability. Consider the following interaction.

> In discussing his school adjustment, the consultant asked a young man if he was a good student. The adolescent responded that he was not and added that he was lazy and not motivated. When asked if he were capable of being a good student, he said no again and offered the opinion that he is "not that smart." The interviewer asked him if he had ever been evaluated and he said, "you mean an IQ test." The young man said that he had been tested and that he had an IQ of 42. The consultant told him that if he in fact had an IQ of 42, he would not be able to sit up in the chair and carry on a conversation and that someone would be feeding him in a bed. The young man laughed and stated his IQ was 113 and in the High Average range. However, he said that the test was 2-1/2 years ago. The interviewer asked if his IQ had gone down since then and the adolescent said he thought it had.

Setting aside the game-playing nature of this interaction, this vignette illustrates this young man's poor opinion of himself.

Hobbies, Interests, and Career Goals

Following questions about school, the next questions are about specific interests and hobbies. This can be valuable in developing suggestions and recommendations for teachers to follow in the classroom to help motivate the young man and reengage him in the educational process. For example, a number of years ago the consultant interviewed a particularly defiant and oppositional young man who was outspoken in his criticism of school and was firm in his refusal to do any work. He felt school was a waste of time, a familiar and frequent comment. However, unlike many young men who demean school as a transparent cover for their lack of success, effort, and/or ability, it was apparent that he was bright and highly motivated. It turns out that he had a singular interest in lobster fishing and any academic pursuit unrelated to that vocation did not interest him. Based on what he learned about the young man's interests in the interview, the consultant suggested to the teachers that they design their curriculum, to the extent that they could, around his interest in lobster fishing. This changed his attitude. He became more attentive and engaged in school. He used his time at home on the weekends to build lobster pots and a boat. After he completed the program, he became a successful lobster fisherman.

Talking about interests is one of the few safe topics for delinquents. "Hanging with my friends" is the most common response to a question of: "When you are at home and can do what you want to do, how do you like to spend your time?" This is followed closely by interests in sports, music, and, somewhat surprisingly, art. A lot of the delinquents have indicated they like to draw. As noted earlier, the "hanging with my friends" response opens the door to questions about drug use. Excessively guarded youngsters, however, are often not any more responsive to questions on this topic than they are to any other topics.

The response to questions about career goals is extremely variable depending on the age of the delinquent. Youngsters at the lower end of the age range of our population (13–14 years) often have no idea what they want to do. Older youngsters may have a clearer idea, but often their goals and plans appear unrealistic. For example, young men interested in sports, particularly basketball or football, may talk about becoming a professional athlete and playing in the NBA or NFL even though they may have never played on an organized team. It is sometimes difficult to tell if their goals and descriptions of their athletic accomplishments represent reality or fantasy. One resident claimed that he had been the starting point guard on his high school varsity basketball team when he was in the ninth grade. He complained that being in the program "cost me an NCAA scholarship" because he had been scouted by Duke University in his junior year. When the interviewer pointed out that being scouted was no guarantee of being offered a scholarship, he accepted it gracefully.

When a youngster with a poor academic history expresses an unusually high achievement goal based on an interest, a useful follow-up question is to ask if he is aware of what the educational and training requirements to achieve that goal. For example, a young man who likes animals may express the desire to become a veterinarian. Another young man with similar interests may say that he wants to work in a pet store and eventually own his own business. One youngster, who was particularly interested in snakes, expressed the desire to become a "herpetologist." A surprisingly large number of young men indicate that they would like to become counselors, residential staff workers in programs like Ocean Tides or in youth prisons, or work in law enforcement. They express the belief that their own experiences on the streets could benefit them in helping other youngsters avoid a life of crime.

Prior Treatment

When a youngster reveals that he has been having difficulty for a while, it is a good idea to ask if his family ever took him to see a counselor. This is a delicate and potentially toxic subject, because many of these young men have negative attitudes about counseling or psychotherapy and contempt for any mental health professional. One young man indicated that he saw a psychiatrist once "for 15 minutes and he wanted to put me on medication for being bipolar." When the interviewer asked him why the doctor thought he was bipolar, the boy replied: "Because I just sat there and didn't answer his questions." It is difficult in many cases to obtain accurate information. Youngsters report that they cannot remember the name of the counselor, the counselor's professional identity, the duration and frequency of the treatment, or where they received the treatment. Occasionally, a delinquent will indicate that he has experienced prior counseling that was genuinely helpful, but this is the exception rather than the rule.

Youngsters with a history of suicidal behavior or aggressive behavior toward others may have been hospitalized in a psychiatric hospital. Detailed questions about when and where the hospitalization occurred, the reasons for it, and the youngster's reaction to the experience are important questions to ask, although they may not be answered in an informed manner. Asking about this can help to identify important behavior, such as prior suicide attempts, that the youngster would not otherwise bring up or acknowledge. It is important to always ask if the youngster has been on any medications or is currently on medication. If medication has been used, inquire if the young man knows the name or type of medication, why it was prescribed, and whether or not it helped. Answers to these questions vary from "I don't know" or "I can't remember" to a detailed and accurate description of the medication and prescribed dosage.

Emotional Responsiveness

One of the reasons that young men get in trouble is because they act before they think. They are quick to respond to emotional arousal and act impulsively. In plain language, they have a "short fuse." As a result, their interpersonal relationships may be characterized by excessive friction, conflict, and hostility. For instance, one resident, who had been charged with resisting arrest, claimed that the police had thrown his mother and pregnant cousin to the ground when they tried to intervene. This angered him and, in his own words, "I took down five cops." Eventually, he was overpowered and brought to the police station where, according to him, the police were throwing chairs at him. "I was not going to stand for that, so I threw the chairs back at them."

It is important to assess the extent of the delinquent's impulsivity, his awareness of it, and willingness to acknowledge it. This is important in terms of treatment planning and prognosis for success. If this issue is addressed directly and in a matter-of-fact and nonjudgmental manner by the interviewer, the adolescent is more likely to describe his emotional reactivity with accuracy and candor. Often, youngsters will not respond to open-ended questions about their anger. Asking what makes them angry may result in an "I don't know." If this is the case, it is helpful to ask specific and pointed questions, such as: "What if someone calls you a name or teases you?" "What if someone said something bad about your mother or family?" If the young man still does not respond, the interviewer can create an "as-if" situation by saying to the youngster:

"If I really wanted to make you mad, and I don't, what would I have to say or do?" By concretizing the situation and making it very specific, this increases the likelihood of getting a response. Specific follow-up questions involve whether the young man is quick or slow to anger. For example, the interviewer may ask: "When you lose your temper, does it happen quickly or are you more likely to do a slow burn?" Furthermore, what does the young man do once he is angry? Does he yell, hit others, punch walls, take a walk, or do something else to express his anger? Finally, how long does it take for him to calm down? One technique that an interviewer can use to stimulate further discussion of this topic is self-deprecating humor. For example, the interviewer may comment that if the young man were to get mad enough to hit an old man like him, the boy might kill or seriously harm him. This can elicit a laugh, lessen the tensions, and, more important, encourage the delinquent to discuss issues he might otherwise avoid.

In trying to assess a youngster's emotional responsiveness, the consultant has noticed that caution, guardedness, and lack of insight tend to be among the most frequent responses. Many of these youngsters are not psychologically minded and find it difficult to describe what they are feeling. For instance, when one young man was asked about the impact of his parents' divorce on him, the boy said: "I didn't cry." In response to the interviewer's comment that he sounded like he was avoiding something, the boy added: "You have to move on." Occasionally, a youngster will express insight or self-awareness. For example, one young man described how his mother had a boyfriend that he liked and generally got along with. One day they had an argument just as the boyfriend was leaving. He was killed in an accident. In discussing this incident, the young man said that he felt bad about it and stated: "Come to think of it, that's when a lot of my troubles started." Another young man, who acknowledged his bad temper, exhibited subtle but observable changes in his posture and eyes as he described his problems with anger. When the interviewer mentioned this to him, the young man commented: "Yeah, my eyes got bigger, didn't they?" He related that he continues to have problems controlling his aggression, even after a considerable amount of anger management training. In his own words: "I'm fine when I am in (anger management) class, but when I am in a situation, it doesn't work." Finally, a depressed youngster, in response to questions about past suicidal ideation or behavior, stated: "I'm sad, but I'm not crazy. I would never do anything to hurt myself."

Peer Relationships

This is a topic that delinquents may or may not be willing to discuss openly. Delinquents have a subculture, usually consisting of other delinquents, and may have an alienated, suspicious, and hostile view of the adult world. Their friendships provide a sanctuary from adults, who they often perceive as intrusive, controlling, and "the enemy." They may be reluctant to talk about their friends out of loyalty or a fear of betraying them. Offering information might be considered as a way of getting their friends into trouble.

A particularly troublesome and delicate area to explore is gang membership. This is often sacred ground. Asking about gang membership runs the risk of completely shutting down the young man so that getting any other information becomes difficult. The interviewer has to weigh the relative advantages of pursuing this topic. The young man's initial reaction often gives a clear signal about whether or not this subject is worth pursuing. Despite the youngster's reluctance, it is important to ask about friendships in order to assess his capacity for relating to others, his level of psychosocial development, his proficiency in forming interpersonal relationships, and whether or not the youngster has a peer support system. Sometimes, youngsters talk openly about their friends and boast about their accomplishments or misdeeds. They take pride in bragging about their mutual exploits. In addition to providing useful information about their peer relationships, this can give valuable insight into their capacity for empathy and feeling close to others.

Sexual Experience

The young men that the consultant has interviewed vary in their sexual experience from naive and inexperienced to being fathers of one or more children to being convicted sex offenders. In most cases, the subject of sex is usually explored in the context of a youngster's interests and peer relationships described earlier. Some, but not all, are sexually promiscuous. Actually, a surprising number of delinquents have indicated that they have little or no sexual experience. The interviewer asks if the young man has a girlfriend, and, if so, how long they have been going out and the seriousness of the relationship. If the young man is sexually active, the consultant asks if he has fathered any children. Sometimes this information comes up spontaneously without having to ask. There can be considerable variability in how delinquents respond to questions in this area. Even if they have considerable sexual experience, they may be reluctant to talk about it because they do not know socially acceptable language for describing their behavior. They only know "street language" and are embarrassed to use that in the presence of the interviewer. Discussions of sexuality can reveal unexpected and sometimes surprising aspects of the young man's personality that are not related to sexual activity per se. For example, the consultant has talked with shy young men with restricted social development who did not have many friends or acquaintances, and was surprised to learn that they were involved in long-term relationships. Their participation in these relationships indicated qualities of loyalty and commitment that were not otherwise apparent. Similarly, some young men who are already fathers reveal a sense of responsibility, duty, and desire to be successful in this role that they do not show in other areas of their lives. They often talk about wanting to be good fathers and prevent their children from having lives like their own.

Even in an era of supposed sexual enlightenment, most delinquents are reluctant to discuss homosexual feelings or behavior. This is a very difficult topic, even for adjudicated sexual offenders who have been charged and convicted of sexual offenses with same-sex victims. Even young men who have had overt homosexual experiences or have prostituted themselves often deny a homosexual orientation. They may explain their behavior in terms of making easy money or having a passive role in the relationship. There is a high level of denial and rationalization. In an all-male residential program, sexual offenders are subject to scapegoating and verbal or physical harassment by other residents. For the sake of their own protection, sexual offenders are instructed not to identify the true nature of their charges. This may contribute to their reluctance to acknowledge any homosexual feelings. Although the consultant has found that the delinquent subculture tends to be homophobic, he has also interviewed some youngsters who welcomed the opportunity to acknowledge and discuss conflicted feelings about sex.

This topic should be approached tactfully, but directly. The interviewer should be alert to cues or comments from the young man that might provide an opening for questions. Although open-ended questions are a useful way to begin, it is usually necessary to ask specific questions to counter any evasiveness on the part of the delinquent. Nonverbal cues, such as changes in posture, voice tone, or frequency in speech can indicate discomfort and potentially useful areas to pursue. Discussion of sexual behavior may provide indications of previously undetected significant issues, such as prior sexual or physical abuse. It is best to ask about prior abuse in a matter-of-fact and direct manner. For example, questions such as: "Has anyone ever touched you in a way that made you feel uncomfortable?" may open the door to self-disclosure.

Identifying Strengths and Competencies

Although diagnostic or assessment interviews often focus on psychopathology or problems, it is a youngster's unique abilities, strengths, and competences that provide the building blocks for successful treatment. The most important purpose of the assessment interview is to elicit information that will be useful in developing an effective and viable plan for rehabilitating the youngster. The young man's competencies provide the foundation for designing an individualized treatment plan that builds on existing strengths. The interviewer may have to look in unexpected or unlikely places, such as the young man's prior criminal behavior, to uncover these strengths. Prior work and school experiences may suggest a pattern of failures or lack of abilities, but their success in their criminal pursuits may reveal talents. On more than one occasion the consultant has been impressed by the sophisticated business acumen of young men in the drug trade. Although their grades in math may not have suggested much ability, their skill in measuring product, estimating costs, and pricing strategies indicated considerable skill in practical mathematics. Exploring a delinquent's crimes in detail can provide revealing information about his intelligence, problem-solving skills, organizational abilities, leadership, perseverance, motivation, and other qualities, which, if redirected, could be valuable in rehabilitation. Sometimes young men reveal that they have been involved in criminal activities for which they have not been charged or apprehended. This suggests that they were able to exercise enough skill and intelligence in committing their crimes to avoid detection and arrest.

Confidentiality in Interviewing

As in all work related to counseling and rehabilitation, confidentiality is a central and important issue. However, in working with court-adjudicated delinquents in which there are established violations of the law, the issue of confidentiality in assessment interviews is a particularly sensitive issue. In the context of evaluating and interviewing youngsters in a residential rehabilitation facility, confidentiality has to be separated into two categories: confidentiality between the agency and the "outside world" and confidentiality within the agency. In the first case, guidelines for confidentiality are clear, straightforward, and in keeping with the traditional views of protection of client rights. As a state-licensed and funded child care facility, the information on particular youngsters and their families is held in the strictest confidence and is made available only with signed releases of information. The agency has a legal and professional obligation to respect the privacy of the client and keep all information confidential.

The issue of confidentiality within the agency is potentially more problematic. As it is important for staff to share pertinent information in order to develop and maintain an effective treatment program, residents are informed when they enter the program that there is no confidentiality among staff members. Staff members are encouraged to avoid getting into situations where youngsters attempt to restrict staff from disclosing or sharing specific information. This is essential in preventing youngsters from manipulating staff or playing one staff member against another. At the same time, it is important to use discretion and good judgment.

Not all staff members have the same relationships with the youngsters and are not equally likely to become aware of sensitive information. For example, the social services counselors that are responsible for individual and family counseling have much greater access to certain kinds of personal information than do the teachers or residential staff. Similarly, in conducting an assessment or evaluation interview, the interviewer is likely to become more familiar with certain issues both by virtue of the interview and the reviewing of records of prior assessments and treatment. Generally, in presenting the purpose of the interview, the consultant does not mention confidentiality unless the youngster specifically asks. Typically, this rarely comes up in the interview. When it does come up, it is usually with regard to a particular question or topic.

Responding to requests for confidentiality is a complex and tricky issue to resolve. As a consultant to the program, it is the interviewer's professional obligation to do as complete, detailed, and accurate assessment as he can and to include all pertinent information in a written report. This is particularly important because the consultant will not be doing follow-up treatment in the form of individual psychotherapy or counseling with the youngster. At the same time, establishing a trusting relationship is the basis for obtaining sufficient information to complete the assessment to contribute to future counseling that will be provided by other staff. Some residents will not disclose important or salient information if they know that this information will not be kept in confidence. This creates a potential conflict between allegiance to the program and its policies and to the individual youngster. When this occurs, the interviewer will remind the youngster of the program policy of non-confidentiality that he agreed to when he entered. The interviewer will then explore with the adolescent the reasons why the youngster wants the information kept confidential. Following this, the interviewer will make a judgment and inform the client of his decision. As a general guideline, the consultant will keep certain information confidential if it has no direct relation to the youngster's charges, no direct bearing on his treatment, and is no threat to the safety or welfare of the young man or anyone else.

The area in which this issue is most likely to come up is in the discussion of the youngster's charges. Often there are discrepancies or inconsistencies in the descriptions the delinquent provides of both his current and prior charges. For example, if a young man reports that he has been charged and convicted of three burglaries, the interviewer will ask him how many he actually committed in distinction to how many he was charged with. If the youngster has in fact committed more than he was charged with, often the youngster will answer this directly, often with pride. However, some youngsters are fearful that if they reveal more information, this could lead to adverse consequences, such as a longer sentence. In this instance, the interviewer will respect the request for privacy and not push further. As the primary purpose of an assessment interview is to form impressions about the delinquent's current psychological functioning and to identify issues that are important for future treatment and education, it is more important to establish a trusting relationship than to alienate the young man by violating his trust or pushing for information that he is not comfortable in revealing. There is often considerable information in the youngster's file that can be obtained after the interview. In fact, particularly guarded or cautious youngsters may tell the consultant that he can "look it up in my file."

Assessing Suicide

All staff members at Ocean Tides have had in-service training in how to notice clues about suicidal ideation in the comments, written work, or behavior of the residents. Any suggestion of possible suicidal thinking is an automatic referral for an immediate assessment by the consulting psychologist. The evidence that this is a successful strategy is provided by the fact that no young man in residence has ever successfully committed suicide, although there have been several that have done so after either completing the program or leaving it. Although all youngsters who undergo the initial interview are screened for suicide, any youngster referred for an evaluation because of suspicion of suicidal thinking receives a more detailed and specific evaluation for suicidal risk. As Shea (1999, pp. 10–11) notes: "The art of suicide assessment is composed of three tasks: (1) gathering information related to the risk factor for suicide, (2) gathering information related to the patient's suicidal ideation and planning, and (3) the clinical decision making that is subsequently applied to these two databases." Shea (1999) indicates that most of the attention has been given to the first and third factors and less attention has been paid to the practical art of assessing suicidal ideation and planning itself. This is the most important area for the clinician to assess. Although it is beyond the scope of this chapter to discuss this topic in the depth it deserves, the reader is directed to Shea's (1999) excellent book, *The Practical Art of Suicide Assessment*.

Ending the Interview

Although there is no set pattern to ending the interview, the consultant usually asks the youngster what he would like to accomplish in the program. If the resident has any specific or general goals, the consultant will ask how the program could help the resident to attain these objectives. Usually, the responses to this are so vague or nonexistent that the information is not helpful. Even when a resident provides a specific response, additional questioning can lead to a dead end. For example, in talking with one young man who had been articulate and responsive during the interview, the interviewer asked the boy how his individual counseling was coming along. Although he indicated that he liked and respected his counselor and that they got along well, the young man said that the counseling was not going well. Puzzled, the consultant asked why. The young man responded that his counseling sessions were on Tuesdays and Tuesday was his "bad day." He proceeded to state that he had been born on a Tuesday and provided a whole litany of "bad things" that had occurred in his life, all on Tuesdays. When the interviewer asked the young man if he would like him to talk to his counselor about changing his appointments to a different day, he said, "No." When asked why not, the boy answered: "It won't make any difference." This is an example of the kinds of contradictions and inconsistencies that can make these young men both frustrating and interesting to interview.

The consultant almost always ends the interview by telling the young man that he has enjoyed talking with him (unless, of course, he has not enjoyed it), thanking him for taking the time to talk with him, wishing the young man good luck in the program, and offering to shake hands.

Writing a Report

After concluding the interview, the final remaining task is to write a summary report that will be included in the resident's file. This report is available to all staff, including teachers, social services counselors, and residential staff. The report includes a summary of important relevant information, such as the resident's behavior during the interview, his family background, his charges, his substance use, his school history, interests and career goals, any prior treatment, the interviewer's impressions of his current personality and cognitive functioning, a diagnosis, and recommendations for treatment. The prevailing attitude in writing the report is that it should be clear, concise, accurate, and written in nontechnical language that is devoid of professional jargon. The goal is to provide the reader with a clear and descriptive word picture of the person the being evaluated. As previously noted, the range of responsiveness to the interview varies from extremely guarded and nonresponsive to highly self-disclosing and articulate, therefore the reports vary accordingly in the amount of information they contain. Appendix C contains four sample reports that reflect some of the variation in evaluation interviews.

CONCLUSIONS

In attempting to assess delinquents by interviewing them, the interviewer is usually "walking a tightrope." No matter how skillful or sensitive the interviewer may be in asking questions, there is always the risk of alienating the youngster and having him close up or remain silent. Attempts to establish rapport may be met with silence or withdrawal. Positive comments, compliments, or traditional relationship enhancement skills might elicit disdain, contempt, or other negative reactions. It can be a frustrating and trying experience for the interviewer. The person conducting the interview should recognize that the interview process is a delicate balance that can be easily, suddenly, and unexpectedly upset. Although proceeding with caution and tact is sometimes successful, at other times boldness, directness, and an unconventional approach can yield better results. It is important to recognize that many delinquents approach the interview from an adversarial stance. Respecting their position, no matter how disagreeable it may be, is essential for any success. A successful interview is defined by the types and amount of information revealed that is useful for treatment and rehabilitation. Specifically identifying positive attributes or skills that can be honed and redirected is especially beneficial.

REFERENCES

Geffner, R. A., Igelman, R. S., & Zellner, J. (2003). Introduction: Children exposed to interparental violence: A need for additional research and validated treatment programs. In R. A. Geffner, R. S. Igelman, & J. Zellner (Eds.), *The effects of intimate partner violence on children* (pp. 1–10). New York, NY: The Haworth Maltreatment & Trauma Press.

Hoge, R. D. (2008). Assessment in juvenile justice systems. In R. D. Hoge, N. G. Guerra, & P. Boxer (Eds.), *Treating the juvenile offender* (pp. 54–75). New York, NY: Guilford Press.

Huxley, A. (1932). *Brave new world.* London, England: Chatto and Windus.

Kagan, R., & Schlosberg, S. (1989). *Families in perpetual crisis.* Albany, NY: W. W. Norton.

Orwell, G. (1933). *Down and out in Paris and London.* London, England: Victor Gollancz Ltd.

Orwell, G. (1945). *Animal farm.* London, England: Secker and Warburg.

Orwell, G. (1949). *Nineteen eighty-four.* London, England: Secker and Warburg.

Salekin, R., & Alexander, B. K. (1991). Cocaine and crime. In A. S. Trebach & K. B. Zeese (Eds.), *New frontiers in drug policy* (pp. 105–111). Washington, DC: Drug Policy Foundation.

Shea, S. A. (1999). *The practical art of suicide assessment: A guide for mental health professionals and substance abuse counselors.* New York, NY: John Wiley.

Sobell, L. G., & Sobell, M. B. (2008). *Motivational interviewing strategies and techniques: Rationale and examples.* Retrieved from http://www.nova.edu/gsc/forms/mi_rationale_techniques.pdf

Sykes, G. M., & Matza, D. (1957). Techniques of neutralization: A theory of delinquency. *American Sociological Review, 22*(6), 664–670.

West, D. J., & Farrington, D. P. (1973). *Who becomes delinquent?* London, England: Heinemann.

CHAPTER 9

Stem the Tide: Case Histories

This chapter consists of six case histories of boys who resided at Ocean Tides. The information was culled from their files, the clinical consultant's interviews with the boys when they were in residence, and aftercare information. Their names have been changed to protect their identities, and permissions to include their stories in this chapter were granted where possible. These cases were selected to provide a sampling of the Ocean Tides boys; their backgrounds, personal, and psychological hurdles; and the outcome of their experience at Ocean Tides.

CASE 1: A STUDY IN CONTRADICTIONS

Ken was an 18-year-old Asian young man who was born in Laos and moved to the United States with his family when he was an infant. When he entered the Ocean Tides program, his family included his mother; stepfather; older brother, aged 19 years; and a 16-year-old younger brother. The older brother was residing with his biological father out of state. Ken's charges were possession of cocaine, assault on a police officer, resisting arrest, discharging a firearm in a compact area, malicious damage, and carrying a 9-mm pistol without a license.

In an apparent gang-related incident, a group of Asian boys had fired shots at a van belonging to a group of Latino boys. An eyewitness identified Ken as one of the shooters. He maintained his innocence and alleged that his younger brother did the actual shooting. Ken was arrested and released. Police were called a second time to the area of Ken's home after a report came in of shots fired. The same vehicle involved in the first incident was circling the area. A police officer explained to Ken that he had just been arrested and released only a half-hour earlier and now the police were called a second time. He instructed Ken to go back into his house and remain there, and that is when Ken told the officer to "go fuck yourself" and that he was going to hang out all he wanted. The police officer walked Ken across the street to his mother and told his mother to keep him inside or else he was likely to be arrested again. As the officer was explaining this to the mother, Ken started yelling at the officer and threatening him. Ken called him a "tough guy" and stated the he was going to "kick his ass." The police officer told him several times to "calm down and go inside." Ken kept yelling at the officer and continued to become more agitated and threatening. Then he took several quick steps toward the officer with his fist balled and raised. The officer had to grab him and wrestle him to the ground, and with the help of a second officer, subdued him. It took several minutes to restrain him. During this process, Ken continued to fight, kick, and struggle.

When the family first came to the United States, Ken lived with his mother and biological father in another state. His mother was forced to flee to another state for her personal safety. Ken's father had a substance abuse problem (alcohol); was a womanizer and gambler; and beat his wife. He also was emotionally and physically abusive to Ken and his brothers. Ken's mother divorced him and, as a result, she became an outcast in the Laotian community and felt alone and ashamed. After his parents divorced, Ken was reunited with his mother in her new location on the West Coast. By that time, she was involved with another man whom she married in the Lao tradition. Ken was able to form a good relationship with his new stepfather and view him as a positive role model. The stepfather had a physical handicap that severely limited his mobility and prevented him from being able to work. Ken's mother worked at a factory job in order to support herself and her husband.

It was there on the West Coast where Ken became gang involved and lost a number of close friends through imprisonment or fatal shootings. Ken was also shot as a result of gang-related activities. Subsequently, he moved back to the Midwest to live with his biological father. Unfortunately, his father had not changed and his drinking had become even worse. Ken met a girl and they had a daughter. Because he continued to have difficulties, Ken and his girlfriend moved again to Rhode Island where his mother had taken up residence.

After Ken got into trouble with the law again, his girlfriend and daughter moved back to the Midwestern city where they had met. With the assistance of his mother, Ken found a full-time job and helped support the family. His mother was frequently called away from her work to deal with Ken and his younger brother and the troubles they often encountered. In the Laotian culture, children are expected to take care of their parents when they are grown, so Ken was conflicted between acting out as a teenager and taking on the role of the responsible adult in the family. He tended to worry about things over which he had no control. Ken thought that he could not be a good son if he was unable to ensure that his mother was happy and comfortable.

He dropped out of school 2 years prior to being incarcerated in order to work and help support the family. As his mother did not speak English, it was left to Ken to help negotiate with community systems and services. While incarcerated, he felt a sense of frustration because he was not home to help his mother deal with her many problems, particularly his younger brother who challenged his mother's authority by engaging in several acts of delinquency.

Ken had a psychological evaluation while in detention at the Rhode Island Training School. The psychologist described Ken as a youngster who subjugated his personal desires in an effort to accommodate the wishes of others, particularly his family. Although calm on the outside, Ken experienced intense inner conflict between his roles and needs. His inability to resolve this internal struggle resulted in anxiety, feelings of opposition, and anger. He felt responsible for other people's happiness and tried to meet the needs of others. When unsuccessful, he was disappointed and felt incompetent. Ken perceived his biological father as an abusive and demanding perfectionist that he could never satisfy. The resulting discomfort led to distrust of his self and others. He was lonely and depressed. Ken feared bringing shame on his mother, the only supportive figure in his life, and being abandoned by her. His preoccupation with fulfilling his perception of his mother's needs interfered with his identity formation. Ken had little coherent sense of self. Although he desired academic success, he did not feel as though he could find the resources to make this happen. Ken's skepticism coupled with his harsh, punitive view of the world placed him at risk for acting out in ways that were self-destructive.

Contrary to what one might expect based on his charges, his aggression toward the police, and the clinical report, Ken did not have any adjustment problems at either the training school or at Ocean Tides. At the training school, the staff described him as a role model for other youths due to his positive behavior and stability. He was an excellent student in class and successfully passed his high school equivalency examination. At Ocean Tides, the goals for Ken's individual treatment were to help Ken focus on his own needs, address his feelings of shame and realize that he is not a bad person, and to help him verbalize his feelings with regard to his painful upbringing. The goals for family treatment were to help the mother and stepfather access community resources and become more self-sufficient, and help the family balance their cultural beliefs with their American lifestyle.

In family counseling at Ocean Tides, Ken's mother was supportive of him. She survived a number of crises, including losing her job and her husband. He moved back to the West Coast. When her husband left, Ken's mother was ostracized in the Laotian community once again because a woman without a partner is considered unfit or incapable of providing for her husband. Ken's mother found another job and a new boyfriend and worked on obtaining her U.S. citizenship. Despite this, Ken felt responsible for his mother and worried about her constantly while in residence during the weekdays at Ocean Tides. He did not like her new partner and felt the boyfriend was taking advantage of his mother's vulnerability. In family meetings, Ken's mother tried to help him understand that she was able to take care of herself and that he should focus on his own goals. Ken also expressed much anger toward his two brothers. They were both in the Midwest and did not keep in contact with their mother, and Ken felt guilty for their actions.

Ken had a successful adjustment to Ocean Tides and was a model resident. He received the award for the best camper after completing a wilderness trip in the summer, won an essay contest, and was awarded scholarship money for college. He maintained good staff and peer relations and completed two semesters at the local community college, earning a 3.78 grade point average out of a perfect 4.00. As a result of his academic success, he gained admission to a small private university in the Midwest and earned a scholarship. Both Ken and his mother were anxious about him moving away and whether or not they could handle the separation. Family counseling addressed these fears and his mother was considering moving to the state where Ken would be going to college. She had an aunt there who told her that the job prospects were good. The goals in both individual and family counseling during the final phase of Ken's residence were to help them deal with feelings about moving away and to help Ken with the practical issues involved in moving to a new location, registering for college, financial planning, and adjusting to college.

Here, in Ken's own words, is a summary of his life that was written in a "hardship essay" while he was a resident at Ocean Tides.

> Hi. Let me introduce myself. My name is . . . I am 17 years old and I have received my GED and have passed two community college courses with a 4.0 average. My ethnic background is Laotian and I have been in the U.S. since I was two years old. It wasn't very easy to have accomplished and get to where I am today. I'm going to give you a brief summary of my life and the obstacles I overcame to make it this far.
>
> I came to the United States when I was 2 years of age. I was raised in a very unhappy marriage between my parents. You could even call my family dysfunctional. My father was a very abusive man, physically and mentally. My mother couldn't speak English so my father was pretty much all I had.
>
> A couple of years have passed and it's pretty much the same in my family. The only difference is that me and my brother were just a little older so we kind of understood about what was going on. We had moved around a lot because my parents wanted to make a new start to try and make things better. They were tired of people instigating and making things worse but it didn't work because my father didn't change. He was an alcoholic and a gambler.
>
> Finally my mother made the decision of leaving. They got a divorce. She made this decision because she couldn't take it anymore and by this time she learned a little English to get by. My father had won the custody battle because in the judge's eye, he was the best parent for me and my brother because he knew how to get to resources better than my mother. In the middle of all this, me and my brother were suffering. I wanted to go to my mother but I couldn't because I had no say in court and I was too young.
>
> When we lived with my father, my older brother got in trouble with the law. He got incarcerated and I had no role model. To me, I lost a part of me because me and my brother were so close.

I lived with the abuse for awhile and when I finally got old enough, I left to live with my mother. I got into a street gang to find a sense of family. That's when my life got more worse. I didn't seem to care about anything. I didn't go to school, just hung around all day.

Then I got incarcerated. It opened up my eyes. I realized that I was very lucky to get charged as a juvenile because if I got charged as an adult, I would've wasted my whole life incarcerated. I took every opportunity they offered me to change and get me ready for when I get out. That's how I got my GED. It made me proud to get my GED. It made me realize that I have the potential to succeed if I really try.

CASE 2: A PREMATURE ENDING

Too many young men at Ocean Tides say that unless they were able to move away from their neighborhoods and get a fresh start, they would be dead before they were 25 years old. The hope is that their prophecy is wrong. Unfortunately, they are sometimes right. The following case depicts the story of a young man from the inner city with an ending that is unfortunately too familiar.

Bill entered Ocean Tides on temporary community placement (TCP) from the Rhode Island Training School, as are most of the boys at Ocean Tides. He had been sentenced for 24 months, 12 months to serve, 12 months suspended, along with supervised probation for 2 years. His charges were possession of marijuana and cocaine. This was his second conviction in less than a year. He previously had been committed to the training school for 12 months, 6 months to serve, 6 months suspended, and probation for 18 months along with restitution for possession of a stolen motor vehicle.

Bill was 17 years old when he entered Ocean Tides. He was a tall, muscular African American young man from a large family. He had four older half-siblings, a twin brother, and a younger sister. His parents were married and had been together for 20 years. Bill's father was at home when he entered Ocean Tides, but was later imprisoned. His mother reported that her husband was living out of state, but he was actually incarcerated at the state prison. In a meeting with his social worker, Bill stated that his mother did not like other people knowing their business so she made up stories. Bill mentioned that he was used to his father being incarcerated and that it was nothing new to hear that his father was back in jail. With the exception of his twin brother and younger sister, everyone in Bill's family had been in trouble with the law at some time during their lives. Bill's mother had been involved with drugs in the past, but she had been clean for a few years. The family lived in the inner city in a three-family house with all levels occupied by a family member. In a home visit, the social worker described the house as "very bare with little in it." His mother reported that sometimes they stayed on the first floor and sometimes on the second floor.

Upon admission to Ocean Tides, Bill described himself as "quiet and funny, good at sports and good at making friends." He said, "I like money and I want to do well in Ocean Tides." He expressed his needs as needing "to get caught up in school and to stay out of further legal trouble." The goals for family treatment were to help Bill increase communication with his parents and develop more trust, and to help Bill share his feelings appropriately. The individual counseling goals were to help Bill learn to make wise decisions and avoid further legal problems, help him learn to think before acting and focus on the consequences of his behavior; encourage him to make better choices in the company of his peers; encourage him to develop positive peer relationships; help him to learn how to be more assertive and say "no" to negative influences; and remind Bill to stay off the streets.

After some initial difficulty, Bill adjusted well to Ocean Tides. He was pleasant and cooperative in counseling and expressed appreciation for what Ocean Tides had done for him. In school, Bill was a hard worker who always completed his assignments and scored well on tests and quizzes. He was doing double credits to catch up with his peers. In residential, his behavior and attitudes were positive. Bill kept his room neat and clean and worked hard on his chores. He tended to keep to himself, although his peer relations were good and his staff relations were excellent. In keeping with the usual protocol, Bill was transferred to one of the extension houses after a few months and began school at the Providence Campus. He was happy to be in the extension house and continued to be a model resident, doing everything that was asked of him. The house director described Bill as one of the most mature residents he had.

While he was still in the main residence, Bill was referred for a psychological evaluation to determine his mental status following a recent shooting and subsequent hospitalization of his best friend. His friend was in critical condition following surgery. Most of the interview focused on the shooting of his friend and the events that preceded it. Bill's mood was serious, worried, and mildly agitated, but he was pleasant, polite, and cooperative, and expressed an eagerness to talk to the psychologist. Bill explained that there were two rival gangs in the inner city. According to him, they were not formal gangs because they did not have colors, "rags," or other identifiable signs. However, they functioned as gangs in terms of their loyalty to each other. His friend had been having dinner with relatives in a restaurant, when one of the rival gang members knocked on the window and called him outside. His friend left the restaurant, expecting to fight, and was shot twice: once in the abdomen and once in the wrist. Bill explained that he heard that one of the bullets hit an artery in the wrist and the doctors were having trouble stopping the bleeding. Bill had not heard the outcome of the surgery and was worried about his friend's health. He speculated that the shooting was probably in retaliation for the killing of a rival gang member several months earlier.

Bill was eager to go home for the weekend so he could visit his friend in the hospital. He was concerned that he would not be allowed to go home because the staff and administration were worried about his safety. To make his point, Bill emphasized that he had gone home every weekend recently without incident and "if anyone wanted to get me, they would have by now." He explained that he appreciated the concern of the staff and knew that they were acting in his best interests. He added that even though he would be completing the program in a month and did not want to jeopardize successful completion, going home to see his friend was his top priority. Bill stated that if not allowed to go home on pass, he would go AWOL; it was that important to him. The consulting psychologist explained to Bill that he would talk with the director of group living about the situation and get back to him. The director of group living explained that Bill had misunderstood their conversation and that he had been told he had the option of staying at Ocean Tides if he did not feel safe. In a subsequent conversation with Bill, he agreed with the director's version of the conversation and felt reassured.

The psychologist's assessment was that Bill's emotional reaction to the situation was appropriate. Although justifiably worried and sad, Bill was not overreacting emotionally, was not clinically depressed, and had no plans to retaliate with violence or aggression. Bill went home for the weekend, visited his friend in the hospital, and returned unharmed and much relieved.

Bill was in aftercare services after being released from the program. He was attending school on a regular basis at the Providence Campus when he was stabbed in a bowling alley on a weekend. After his release from the hospital and his recovery, his attendance at school dropped off significantly. Due to his many absences, Bill was told that he would not graduate in June as originally scheduled. He could return in September for one semester. If he attended regularly and maintained his grades, he would graduate the following January. Bill accepted this plan and stated that he would return to Ocean Tides in September.

Bill never got the chance to return to school. In July, he and a friend were talking in Bill's car when the friend noticed three men walking in the middle of the road toward the car. One of the men was an old rival of Bill's and he had a gun in his hand. As the men approached the car, the assailant lifted his arm and fired directly into the automobile, hitting the windshield. Bill and his friend fled from the car. A bullet grazed Bill's friend in his side while he was running down the street trying to escape a hail of bullets. Bill was not so lucky. He was found dead behind a stockade fence in the rear yard of a neighboring house. An autopsy revealed that he died from a single gunshot wound. A bullet recovered from Bill's chest was fired from the same gun that fired the bullet found in the windshield. Bill's friend and several eye witnesses had identified the assailant. He was apprehended the next day. In a trial, the jury found the assailant guilty of first-degree murder, conspiracy to commit murder, use of a firearm during a crime of violence resulting in death, assault with a dangerous weapon, and possession of a firearm without a license. He was sentenced to consecutive life sentences plus 40 years for Bill's murder and the assault on his friend.

CASE 3: FROM A CHAOTIC FAMILY TO HEROISM

David was a slender Caucasian young man who entered Ocean Tides at age 16 years. He was sentenced to the training school with TCP at Ocean Tides following charges of shoplifting and malicious damage. David had previously been charged with felony assault, simple assault, and malicious damage. The earlier felony assault charge occurred when he threatened his older sister with a knife and a meat cleaver during an argument. He maintained he was not going to hurt her but just wanted to scare her. The simple assault charge was the result of a fight with a peer at school. While playing basketball, David reported that he assaulted the other young male with a stick because he had thrown a brick, a crate, and a stick at him.

David came from a dysfunctional family background characterized by his biological parents' substance abuse, abandonment, and neglect by the biological mother and physical abuse by the father. He was the second oldest of three children, with an older sister and younger brother. David's parents divorced when he was 3 years old. His mother had a history of abusing alcohol and cocaine but had been sober for 5 years prior to David's incarceration. After the divorce, she lost custody of the children to her former husband due to her substance abuse. David was initially placed in a foster home prior to moving in with his father. The family lived in the East but relocated to the Midwest when David was 9 years old so that his father's girlfriend could be closer to her family. The couple eventually broke up and the family returned to the East Coast.

David reported that his father was physically abusive to him and his siblings. He reported an incident in which his father threw a speaker at his brother and another time when his father threw David off the porch into a metal pipe causing a wound that required stitches. The state Department of Social Services investigated this incident and substantiated its occurrence. The investigation revealed that the family was living in the car. The children were not attending school and had head lice. David reported that he and his siblings did not argue or fight during that time because "we were too busy protecting ourselves." After the abuse investigation, David and his siblings were removed from their father's custody and were placed in separate foster homes for about 1 year before being reunited with their mother, who had maintained sobriety and freedom from drugs for 4 years. At the time David entered Ocean Tides, he had not had any contact with his biological father for 3 years. David expressed interest in seeing his father, but his social worker was unable to locate him despite several attempts.

The reunification with his mother did not go smoothly. She was still living with her second husband, whom she divorced after 3 years. The divorce was amicable. Although she and her former husband now lived apart, they remained friends and visited often. David's mother reported an increase in his behavior problems and filed a disobedient petition. David was impatient over little things, was defiant to his mother, and had frequent altercations with his two siblings. His mother reported that he lost his temper easily and this would involve throwing things, damaging property, and swearing. An assessment of the family revealed that the relationship between David and his mother was strained by her resentment that he had problems and by David's failure to be aware of or contain his inappropriate behavior. It appeared that David's mother scapegoated him and focused on him as the problem in the family. She candidly admitted that if David did not improve, she did not want him at home.

David had been hospitalized twice for psychiatric problems. The first admission occurred when he was 12 years old and was precipitated by mood swings, withdrawal, isolation, and aggressive behavior. He said he wanted to die and walked across streets in front of moving traffic in an apparent effort to be hit by cars. At that time he was living with his father and his father's girlfriend. David had difficulty getting along with siblings, peers, and adults. He was impulsive and explosive, and got into a lot of fights. He withdrew to his room, cried, and engaged in self-abusive behaviors, such as hitting himself on the head and banging his head against the walls. He was diagnosed with major depression and oppositional defiant disorder. David was discharged with a prescription for antidepressant medication.

The second hospitalization occurred when he was 15 years old for evaluation of possible depression and concern for suicidal ideation based on statements he had made to his outpatient therapist about wishes to die. There was also concern for possible psychotic process because of visual and auditory hallucinations. David stated that he believed he had good and evil "spirit masters" that were fighting to have control over him. He stated that the evil spirit master was telling him to harm himself. In a subsequent psychological evaluation, David explained that he had been conversing with an "imaginary friend" that he named "Spirit Master." Psychotherapy and medication helped. David explained why he had an imaginary friend as: "I probably needed someone to talk to because at that time I was very alone. I was residing at a foster home. I had no friends and I wasn't with my other siblings. I guess I just needed someone to be with. I don't have him any longer."

Several psychiatric and psychological evaluations suggested that David acted in an impulsive, defiant, and irritable manner in order to ward off his recurring periods of depression and anxiety. His poor impulse control affected his ability to use good judgment in social situations or to understand his behavior. David acted impulsively and angrily when he was confronted with emotionally charged situations and was overwhelmed by his feelings. Consequently, he was at risk for aggressive and impulsive behavior when confronted or criticized. Psychological testing indicated that David had average intelligence.

Prior to coming to Ocean Tides, David attended a special school for behaviorally disturbed students and was enrolled in an outreach project run by an outpatient nonprofit social services agency. He cooperated with the program, attended school regularly, and achieved good grades and awards for his performance. David did not display any of the oppositional, defiant, or aggressive behavior in school that he exhibited at home. His family relationships improved. He followed his mother's rules and attempted to make positive changes. His mother worked hard to see the changes and acknowledged David's improved behavior. However, when school ended for the summer, his behavior regressed. He stopped following the house rules and was late for curfew. His mother expressed concern that he might be getting into trouble in the community.

David had an inconsistent adjustment to the Ocean Tides program. He vacillated between doing well at times and accumulating a lot of sanctions at other times for noncompliant behavior both in school and in residence. He displayed an unusual sense of humor at times and exhibited a constant need for attention. David tended to pick on some of the other residents and his behavior could be annoying. His behavior in school was also inconsistent. Sometimes he would refuse to do work for certain teachers. David formed a close relationship with several of the residential counselors and talked about them as "father figures." These relationships were a very important part of his treatment. David's treatment plan emphasized learning better anger management and impulse control.

In an evaluation with the consulting psychologist, David talked in detail and at length about the physical abuse he had experienced at the hands of his father. He reported that his father drank alcohol every day and was abusive to him and his younger brother, but not to his sister. He stated that his father beat him every day and sometimes twice a day. The abuse included his father's hitting him with his fist. On days when his father drank more, the beatings intensified. David adamantly denied using marijuana, alcohol, or any other drugs, although there was contradictory information in his file that indicated he had experimented with both marijuana and alcohol. Similarly, he denied that he had anger or impulse control problems except with his brother. Although David looked depressed and anxious, he did not report any clinically significant symptoms of either disorder.

David successfully completed the program. During the second half of his treatment, he moved to a house and did well there. He related well to both staff and peers, showed a positive attitude, and was responsible in doing his chores and keeping his room clean. After completing the program, he continued at the Providence Campus where he did well academically. As part of his studies, David volunteered as a teacher's aide at an elementary school and his evaluation reports were very good.

Thirteen years after completing the Ocean Tides program, David, at 29 years of age, was killed in Afghanistan. As a sergeant in the National Guard for 11 years, he died after saving a 3-year-old Afghan boy from being hit by an armored vehicle. Witnesses reported that several Afghan children were in the path of the convoy. David saw the young boy trying to retrieve an item on the road, removed him to safety, and was hit and killed by the vehicle. David was awarded the Bronze Star posthumously. His parents, fiancée, and three young children survived him. David died a hero. At a memorial service, he was remembered as having "the courage of a warrior" and "the heart of a father."

CASE 4: TURNING HIS LIFE AROUND

Enrique was Latino and entered Ocean Tides when he was 17 years old. He was the youngest of five children with three older sisters and one brother. The parents and all of the children were born in Mexico to married parents. His mother came to the United States with three of the children and left two in her parents' care in Mexico. They had been in America for 11 years when Enrique was charged. There was no contact with the father since the family left Mexico, but the mother remained in regular and close contact with her two daughters who remained there.

Enrique was charged with robbery, assault, and trespassing. This was his first criminal charge. In an interview with the consulting psychologist, he explained that all three charges occurred on the same day. Enrique denied that there was an assault. He said that he and a friend saw another young man walking with a girl and a dog. This young man was wearing Enrique's gang colors. When he saw Enrique and his friend, he began to run and they chased him. They ended up in a convenience store. Enrique "asked" the victim for his necklace. Although Enrique admitted that he stole the necklace, he denied that any assault occurred. He said the victim lied about it. A fight did occur between Enrique, his friend, and some members of a rival gang, but everyone scrambled away to avoid police detection. They went into a nearby yard and saw a house with an open door. They entered to hide. Enrique thought that a neighbor saw them, which is why they were charged with trespassing. He said that he was originally sentenced to serve 3 years: one in the training school and two in the adult prison. However, his public defender was able to get the sentence reduced to 1 year to serve, 1 year suspended, and 1 year of probation. Enrique spent 5 weeks in the training school prior to entering Ocean Tides.

Enrique admitted to heavy marijuana use and reported that he smoked about seven "blunts" every day. He stopped using marijuana when he was incarcerated and had not smoked since that time. Although he did admit to smoking a joint on an occasional basis, like when he was at a party, he no longer used it on a regular basis. He would drink alcohol occasionally at parties, too, but did not smoke cigarettes or use any other drugs.

Enrique impressed the consulting psychologist as sincere, likeable, outgoing, and good natured. However, beneath that pleasant surface was an emotionally labile young man with a short temper who was easily angered. He was a large boy, muscular and strong, and he could seriously hurt someone. He was aware of that and unlike some of the other residents he did not use his size or strength to either intimidate or bully other smaller residents. On the contrary, Enrique described himself as a peacemaker and someone who tried to bring people together.

School had been a problem for Enrique since he moved to the United States. He had to start school over because the system here was so different from what he had in Mexico. Prior to coming to Ocean Tides, Enrique had completed the eighth grade but had trouble adjusting to high school. He attended two public high schools, and was "thrown out" of the first and found it difficult to concentrate and pay attention at the second because the other students talked a lot in class, so he stopped going.

Enrique was formally a member of the "OCG" or Original Cripps Gang, but dropped out because he felt unsupported by them. They never wrote, called, or contacted him when he was in the training school except for one time when they called him on a weekend. They wanted his help with an upcoming fight with a rival gang. Enrique told them in no uncertain terms that he wanted nothing more to do with them. In his own words, "You didn't help me when I needed help, so why should I help you?"

When Enrique entered Ocean Tides, the initial assessment described him as a friendly, respectful, loyal to his friends, and a good worker. The goals for individual treatment were to help Enrique recognize and verbalize how his emotions were connected to the behaviors that led to his charges, to use tutoring and small classroom groupings to develop more effective study skills and improve his academic performance, and to help him develop more effective decision-making skills. The goals for family counseling were to help his mother establish age-appropriate expectations and rules with consistent consequences for Enrique when he was at home on passes, and to verbalize the anger, frustration, and resentment related to financial stress and the limitations for better employment opportunities due to the family's legal status.

Enrique adjusted well almost immediately upon entering the program. He was respected by his peers and well thought of by all staff. He enjoyed recreational activities and was an active participant. Enrique did not receive any sanctions from either residential staff or teachers for misbehavior, a rare occurrence for a resident. In school, he was focused, highly motivated to do well, and a hard worker. His behavior was quiet, but well mannered, respectful, and polite. He impressed his social services counselor as a mature young man that wanted to benefit from his opportunity at Ocean Tides. He expressed a desire to work in the kitchen and worked there regularly. He also worked with the maintenance department and received good reports for his work. Enrique was open and cooperative in counseling and his mother participated in all the scheduled family counseling sessions. He earned double credits (10th and 11th grades) to catch up in school. He was transferred to an extension house in Providence, and won the "Best Student of the Week" award in the first week. He had newfound confidence in his academic skills and decided to stay at the Providence Campus after his release from the program in order to graduate. Enrique's academic success had a markedly beneficial effect on his self-concept. He went from someone with a low opinion of his cognitive abilities, who thought of himself as a failure, to a confident young man eager to continue his education after high school. At one point he returned to both his high schools to show his former teachers his report card because he was so proud of himself. They were pleased and surprised. A former teacher with whom Enrique had a good relationship kidded him and said that he did not think he had it in him to do so well. The teacher admitted he was wrong and asked Enrique "How much do I owe you?" Enrique was pleased with his reception.

Enrique did extremely well during aftercare. He attended school regularly and did very well academically, making all As in his classes during the first quarter. His mother reported that she was pleased with his attitude and behavior at home. He kept all of his appointments with his counselor and remained trouble free in the community. In view of his outstanding record, the governor appointed him to the student seat on the Juvenile Justice Advisory Committee of the Rhode Island Justice Commission. At his court review, the judge ordered the termination of Enrique's aftercare and closed his case as a reward for his outstanding behavior.

In an essay in school, Enrique described his life as follows.

> I am a proud young man of Mexican heritage, and this is my story.
>
> When I was in the seventh grade at OH School, I witnessed two gangs having a rumble in the playground across the street from my school. I left school to watch the fight. As I was watching, I was moved by the loyalty and love the gang members had for each other. One day in mid October, I watched another rumble, and when the losing gang turned and ran for their lives, being chased by the other gang, I was the only one left standing there. The OG (Original Gangsta) from the set came toward me, so I put up my hands, ready to fight. Instead of swinging at me, he asked me what my name was. At first, I stayed quiet, thinking something was up. Then he asked me if I wanted to get down with his gang.
>
> Taken by surprise, my mouth opened, and I said "yes." Soon after, I was being "jumped in" by the gang, the way you become a member. I tried to fight back, but there were too many of them. At the end of getting jumped, as I lay on the

ground, they gave me a hand getting up and said, "welcome to the family young Cuz (cousin)."

The years passed, and I was still a part of the gang. I had earned respect the hard way, and I liked it. I enjoyed the company of my homeboys, but sometimes I like being by myself. In high school, I was known as one of the baddast gang members there. One day, I was snitched out by a rival gang for doing something that, today, I am ashamed of and won't talk about. The cops and principal came looking for me, and caught up to me in my US History class. I was expelled from XX high school for my actions.

I enrolled in XZ High School, and they had good expectations for me, but I still hadn't learned my lesson. I still proudly wore my colors up and down the hallways of XZ High School. Even after getting in trouble and being given a second chance, I broke the rules again by being directly involved in gang-related violence. I was expelled from XZ, and no other school would take me.

Now, I was out of all the public schools in Providence. Shortly after that, a friend of mine (also a gang member) got thrown out of school for the same reason as me. We had a so called "vacation" together. Not too long after, we were both arrested for gang-banging. The judge gave my boy a four month slap on the wrist sentence, but unloaded a shotgun blast of bad news into me. I had to serve a year. Since that day, I've found out who my real friends are. None of my gang "family" wrote to me while I was locked up to see how I was doing, or if I needed anything done. While I was locked up at the Training School, I realized that gang banging wasn't doing me any good, wasn't making my life any better, so I hung it up.

The Training School took my freedom (to be honest, I threw my freedom away by doing the things I had been doing) and tried to play with my life. I surmounted that predicament, and realized I needed to get an education so I could rise above the streets. I could be successful in school once I got my head screwed on straight. Who got in my way and prevented me from succeeding? I was the baddast, remember? Now that energy would get used for good reasons and positive outcomes.

I had heard of the Ocean Tides School, and wanted to look into it. The judge told me it was a good school, and I would be able to do double credits, make up for time I had wasted at my other schools. I jumped at the opportunity to go to OT. It would get me out of the Training School and give me a chance to get something positive accomplished with my life.

I've been at Ocean Tides for over a year now. Once my sentence was up, I chose to stay at OT and finish my high school education. They do good work with kids like me. They helped me realize my potential and feel happy for me when I succeed. I've accomplished some of my goals, made some positive changes in my life. Now, I'm going to be graduating from high school in June of 2006. Whatever comes after that, I know that I'll be better prepared to deal with life in positive ways and maybe be able to help other people make good choices in their lives.

CASE 5: STRUGGLE LEADS TO SUCCESS

Sometimes a young man needs a second chance before he can take the opportunity to turn his life around. The following case is from a resident who completed the program more recently, and it is included as an example of how persistence and the opportunity for a second chance can lead to a positive outcome.

Robert was an African American young man who was born in Liberia, Africa, and moved to the United States with his mother and siblings when he was 3 months old. He never met his father who died while on a job for the United Nations when Robert was 13 years old. Robert had contact with his father by phone calls on a few occasions. He remembers that his mother would often not let him talk to his father and would claim that Robert was not at home when he would be standing right next to his mother while she talked to her husband on the phone. His family included his mother, maternal grandmother, two half sisters (aged 32 and 29 years), a 21-year-old sister and her two children (aged 1 and 2 years), and a 6-year-old half sister. His two older sisters lived independently and one was out of state. The rest of the family lived together in Providence, where they lived since coming to the United States. They moved eight times while living in the same city. Robert was not close with anyone in his family and felt that he could not rely on any of them. They all had their own lives. His mother worked as a home health care aide.

Robert was in residence at Ocean Tides on two separate occasions. He had also been in the training school five times. He was 14 years old the first time and was in the program for 11 months. He had been charged with first-degree robbery, conspiracy, resisting arrest, vagrancy, and assault with the intent to commit robbery. He was sentenced to 2 years of probation; a 1-year suspended sentence; and 6 months of home confinement with an electronic ankle bracelet, restitution, and a no-contact order. Five months later, Robert was held at the training school for charges of disorderly conduct, failure to comply with home confinement, and violating a valid court order. He was sentenced to 2 years of probation with 1 year to serve and 1-year suspension. He was placed at Ocean Tides on TCP.

Prior to entering the program, Robert had done well in elementary and middle school but started to have problems when he entered high school. He had transferred schools several times and had an Individual Education Plan (IEP) to address his academic learning and behavioral needs. He had experimented with marijuana at age 14 years and his mother reported finding an empty alcohol bottle in the home. She also reported that Robert had become increasingly noncompliant at home and would respond aggressively when she would attempt to set limits or implement consequences. Robert had a history of difficulty managing conflict and had a low frustration tolerance. He had many negative peers, could easily be instigated by them to engage in conflict or disruptive behavior, and had difficulty at times taking direction from authority.

During his first stay at Ocean Tides, Robert described himself as quiet and funny, being good at football and basketball, and he admitted he needed to get his life together. He hoped to become a doctor. In his early adjustment, Robert was active in participating but needed to improve his attitude. His behavior changed for the better after the first month. He made good grades in school and worked hard. Robert liked to work independently, but he became extremely frustrated if he did not understand the material. At times he would get off task and engage in negative behavior, such as teasing and instigating fellow students. When corrected, he could become oppositional, angry, and defensive. Shortly after earning his weekend passes, he was picked up by the police for trespassing at a mall because he had a no-contact order for this location from a past disorderly conduct charge.

Robert continued to improve and had better relations with both staff and peers. He was an excellent worker in the kitchen, actively participated in all recreational activities, kept a clean room, practiced good personal hygiene, and did well with his daily chores. He transferred to one of the extension houses in Providence and began school at the Providence Campus. He continued to do well with the staff, but had some difficulties with the other residents. He was easily instigated and could be loud, excitable, impulsive, and immature at times. He continued to do well in school in Providence and earned two awards; "Student of the Week" award and "Hardest Working Student at the Science Fair." He even made the honor roll. Teachers described Robert as a motivated student with a positive attitude toward school. However, his peer relations were still strained and he could anger quickly. His mother initially showed up for family meetings but then canceled many times because of her work and did not participate for months. After she received a letter about the importance of attending family meetings, she showed up more regularly. Individual counseling sessions with Robert focused on helping him learn some techniques to control his temper and he enrolled in the Anger Management Group. Robert's mother reported that he was respectful, had good behavior, and had a good attitude on his weekend passes while he was on the Providence Campus.

Unfortunately, about a month before he was to complete the program, Robert was arrested by Providence police at his house and returned to the training school. The house director reported that he had heard that Robert had been involved in a violent incident where he allegedly robbed and beat up someone. Although Robert was involved with an outpatient family service agency at the time, he picked up additional charges of possession of a stolen motor vehicle, driving without a license, obstruction, and conspiracy. He was placed on TCP at Ocean Tides again.

Robert was 16.5 years old when he entered Ocean Tides for the second time, and that stay went well. He knew what was expected of him and adjusted quickly. Robert was more mature and did well in all phases of the program. In school he worked on making up deficits in reading comprehension, writing, and math computation. Robert responded well to directions and resource services. Although he could get off task occasionally, he was easily redirected. He was polite with staff and appropriate in his interactions with peers. He decided to finish at the Providence Campus and graduate from there. Robert worried that if he returned to public high school there was a good chance he would get into legal trouble again. He did not like talking about his family in counseling and would shut down when the topic was introduced. He considered his godmother more of a resource than his actual mother. His mother worked long hours and even though the social worker talked with her about the importance of supervising Robert, she did not think that she could keep track of him now that he was 17 years old. Robert was also upset that his older sister Angela, who he once considered his best friend, was not there for him. He came to the realization that if he wanted to go on to college, he was going to have to do it on his own.

Robert completed the Ocean Tides program and was released from the residential component. He continued at the Providence Campus and graduated. While attending school, he completed 45 hours of community service at a Neighborhood Ministries after-school program and continued to volunteer there. In that role, he tutored and mentored students, and he was well liked and respected by the staff.

Robert was accepted and offered a grant to attend a private college in Providence. As of this writing, he is a second-year student in good standing. The following is an essay he wrote during his senior year of high school, which is his life story in his own words.

Struggle Leads to Success

Growing up was not easy living in the projects. My mother was a refugee from the war in Liberia who fought to get to the United States so she could provide a better life for her family.

My mom worked many hours at the Nursing Home. As I got older I wanted to be more of a man for myself because to her I was just her baby, but in the neighborhood I was Sunny. I started dealing crack at the age of twelve. I learned to deal very fast. I started feeling like dealing crack was a part of me, or in my blood, like how Michael Jordan was so gifted at basketball. I was bringing in $800.00 a week.

One day I went home after school and my mom was crying. I knew something was really wrong for her to be home during the day. My mother looked at me and said, "Sunny, your father died." All I could think was why? What hurt me the most was that I never got to know him. I never saw him but I would talk to his picture every night wishing he would come to see me. I would hear from him from time to time but at age thirteen it just was not enough. I felt like I was supposed to know this man and he was supposed to raise me to be a man. Maybe he could have stopped me from doing the wrong things but now he was gone.

Once he died I promised myself that I wasn't going to go back to dealing and try and do something positive with my life. I started to play football and basketball for local teams to avoid dealing or being shot in the projects but that didn't last long. I went right back to dealing and my friends and I started to get in trouble together. I ended up going to the Rhode Island Training School on a second-degree robbery charge.

While at the Training School I remember crying in my room knowing that the place was not for me. I started praying to God, hoping he would help me with my situation. At court I was released and placed on home confinement. I was doing okay for a while but again I started dealing knowing full well the risks I was taking. I was arrested again and sent back to the Training School to serve fifteen months on a first degree robbery and felony assault charge. I was still an angry kid but knew I had to make a change. Once I got back on the streets I tried to develop a positive attitude and stay away from all the negativity. Still missing my father and finding it harder and harder to overcome the struggles, I reverted to my old ways and became involved in more serious crimes.

Finding myself in the Training School yet again, I thankfully found myself realizing that the life I was leading had no purpose other than to keep me in jail for a long time or worse, dead. I prayed that at my next court appearance if God could help me to see this through I would do everything I could to become a better, stronger person. In court my lawyer told me the great news: he had gotten me a deal that would send me back to Ocean Tides on temporary community placement and probation until I turned nineteen. I remember feeling so lucky and grateful.

When I got to Ocean Tides I felt like a new person. I had put my past behind me and was ready to move forward. I told myself over and over that I was better than my past. Over the next few months I found myself maturing and knowing that I didn't have to be so cold hearted or mad all the time. I continued to learn more about myself and I was becoming wiser and started seeing my life how I wanted it to be. I set goals for myself to accomplish that would provide me with what I wanted. My motto was to set a goal and once I completed that goal, to set another. I started doing really well and became more humble. It was then that doors started to open for me.

That summer I was placed at a summer job with a program called South Providence Neighborhood Ministries (Louie's Place) working with kids ages 7 and 8. It was something I always want to do. I learned things like how to be more calm and patient, because God only knows what those kids had been through. I knew that I could relate to them in many ways. I fit right in and I loved it. Every morning I would wake up with a smile on my face just knowing I was going to work with those kids. It got to a point when I didn't even care about the money or that I was still at Ocean Tides, I just wanted to see those kids smile.

The summer came to an end and my senior year was starting and I needed a plan. I did an internship at the Ministries; there were fewer kids but the same beautiful smiles. It was there that I decided that I wanted to study counseling and that I wanted to go to college to accomplish it. I did my homework, continued my internship and started applying to colleges like Johnson and Wales and CCRI to major in counseling and psychology. I was taking the necessary steps to succeed. I kept my grades up and presented myself in better ways so that people could see that I came out of the projects and I had some trouble but that was hopefully behind me. You can change as long as you are willing to change. Through all my cold days and rough nights I have come a long way. I have been accepted at Johnson & Wales and am grateful for the opportunity to prove myself.

My plan is to attend Johnson & Wales for four years majoring in counseling and psychology [and] continue my education to earn a master's degree. I would like to work with kids between the ages of twelve and eighteen. I will always work hard and never forget where I came from and what made me who I am today.

My ultimate goal is to be happy, receive my Ph.D., open my own mental health clinic and an all boy's school, marry a beautiful lady, and start a family. I will raise them to believe that they don't have to do wrong. I want them to understand that no matter what, life is a gift and you should always stay strong because struggle leads to success.

CASE 6: A HORATIO ALGER STORY

Carl was a tall, lean, nice-looking, 17-year-old Caucasian young man who came to Ocean Tides for violating his probation on a felony assault charge of discharging a BB gun within the city. He was placed on probation for assault with a dangerous weapon in the public library. Carl said he was provoked by another teenager and swung his backpack, which contained a lock, hitting the victim in the head. The teenager required seven stitches to close the wound. Carl said that he forgot he had the lock in his backpack. He had previous charges of larceny and breaking and entering. Some of his prior thefts involved stealing objects from unlocked cars and from unlocked garages. Carl was also charged with shoplifting items from a department store. His explanation of his most recent charge was that he was shooting at a sign and a woman, "who happened to be standing near the sign," pressed charges. He told different versions of the story at different times. His other explanations were that he was taking the blame for a friend and he was trying to scare the woman, who he claimed was a drug addict.

Carl is very loyal to his friends and said that he would fight with others who threatened them. He was not a member of a formal gang but revealed that he and seven or eight of his buddies called themselves "Dick Heads." They were not well known but would leave their "tag" (graffiti with their name) everyway. Carl carried mace as a weapon. He and his friends had cap guns that they had painted to look like real guns to intimidate gang members so that they would be left alone.

Carl was the oldest of three children born to his biological parents. He had a 15-year-old brother and 12-year-old sister. His parents divorced when Carl was 10 years old after 10 years of marriage due to his father's addiction to heroin and cocaine. His father had a history of verbal and physical abuse against his family that Carl often witnessed. Although his father had attended several residential substance abuse programs over the years, he usually relapsed several months after completing the programs. Despite the divorce, Carl's mother felt a need to continue to care for her former husband. For example, when he was discharged from a treatment program, she let him live in the family's apartment for several months and even paid him to babysit for their youngest child. This particularly annoyed Carl and his brother.

Two years previously when Carl was starting to act up, his mother sent him to live with his father on Nantucket Island. Carl reported that his father was house painting and using and selling drugs at the time. He took care of his father and even provided a sample of his own urine so that his father would have a clean drug screen for his probation officer. After the divorce, the family lost their home and his mother began working two jobs in order to try and support her three children. She had a history of anxiety and depression and had been treated in a psychiatric day program in the past for depression. Carl's mother placed high demands on herself to take care of the family and experienced considerable continuing stress due to financial pressures and her other responsibilities. Although the family members cared greatly for one another, there was frequent conflict, arguing, and yelling.

Carl had several clinical evaluations prior to entering Ocean Tides, including both interview-based assessments and projective testing. The evaluations suggested that Carl was a highly conflicted and impulsive young man who required a great deal of external stimulation in order to keep from being bored. His judgment and impulsive behavior got much worse when he was under stress. He was highly influenced by those around him, especially peers who were getting into trouble. Carl had a great deal of repressed anxiety, anger, and sadness, particularly with regard to his father's substance abuse problems and his mother's continuing struggle with depression and anxiety. He worried about his mother's well-being and felt that she was so stressed out at times that she might commit suicide. Carl was very action oriented and his impulsive style prevented him from controlling his own behaviors easily. He had a good sense of right and wrong but it was not enough to prevent him from engaging in antisocial behavior. His ability to delay gratification was immature for his age. Carl required a lot of structure and feedback in his day-to-day functioning in order to help guide his actions and prevent him from engaging in behavior that would get him into trouble.

The treatment plan for Carl when he entered Ocean Tides involved both family and individual goals. The goals for family counseling were to address the enmeshment of the divorced parents, encourage Carl's mother to place the needs of her children above those of her ex-husband, learn to take care of her own needs, and to plan for her life after her children were grown and leave the home. The goals for Carl's individual treatment were to help him learn to take care of himself, provide an atmosphere of support, help him to not feel overly responsible for caring for his parents, and enable him to separate himself from his family in an appropriate way. Carl was highly motivated to attend college. His treatment plan was designed to help him catch up in school and graduate from high school and to achieve his goal of furthering his education by providing the necessary resources to apply to colleges and obtain financial aid.

When Carl met with the consulting psychologist, he was polite, respectful, and cooperative. He demonstrated good interpersonal skills, communicated clearly, and answered questions completely and openly. He tended to avoid talking about some uncomfortable issues, such as his father's substance abuse, and minimized the seriousness of his charges. Carl demonstrated the social skills necessary to make a good first impression. While he appeared superficially comfortable, there were signs of underlying anxiety, difficulty with controlling his impulses, and the potential for bad judgment and poor decision making when his emotions were aroused. He admitted to occasional use of marijuana and alcohol, but was not a frequent user of either substance. Carl did not show any signs or symptoms of a mood or thought disorder and was not at risk for harming himself or others.

Carl did very well in the program. He made consistent progress in school and participated in all activities. He was a member of the basketball team that won the league championship. He was transferred to an extension house after 6 months and continued to do well there. Carl obtained his driver's license and was able to get a car. This access to transportation enabled him to work delivering pizzas on his weekend passes. He completed a successful section of the culinary arts program and received excellent reports from the teachers of his academic subjects. The only blemish on his record was a single incident in which he had a fight with another resident. Carl talked openly in individual counseling and most of the time was spent on family issues and future plans, including applications for college. Carl stated that he was happy to be at Ocean Tides because it gave him some space from his family and allowed him to pursue his own needs. At the same time, he was able to remain connected to his family. His father moved to Florida and his absence helped the family function better because they did not have to worry about him. His mother's attendance at family counseling sessions was inconsistent, but she participated fully when she came.

Carl successfully completed the program. After his release he continued his education at the Providence Campus of the Ocean Tides School and graduated. He met the goals that he had set for himself by graduating from high school and being accepted to college (Rhode Island College). Carl received several awards at the graduation ceremony, including the Pell Medal for excellence in history, the Family Court Judges' Award, and a scholarship award. His mother attended graduation with other family members but his father did not travel from Florida to attend the ceremony as he had promised he would.

The last sentence of Carl's Termination Report from Ocean Tides states: "He remains a highly motivated young man who has the potential to succeed." This turned out to be a prophecy that came true. Carl founded and is president of a highly successful valet car service that is used by more than 20 high-end restaurants and other businesses in Rhode Island and Southeastern Massachusetts. He is a strong advocate for Ocean Tides and is on the board of directors. As of this writing, he is organizing the first-ever cookout to be held for Ocean Tides alumni and staff.

In the following excerpt taken from an essay submitted for a scholarship competition, Carl described his life.

> Prior to coming to Ocean Tides, I was basically a high school dropout. I was always being suspended for vandalism and fighting. The rest of the time I just didn't bother to attend school. For these reasons, I was failing all my courses. I believe that I was basically just acting out because I was angry about the way things were going at home.
>
> My parents were divorced when I was 8 years old. Until this year, my father was a substance user who spent his life in and out of rehab. My mother, on the other hand, was a hard

worker who tried to provide a good life for my siblings and me. My mother was rarely seen at home because she worked two jobs, however, she continued to encourage us to do our best. Neither of my parents graduated from high school. My mother reached the ninth grade and my father reached the twelfth. I received little education from my parents after the age of six because what they could teach me was limited.

After repeated arrests and suspensions from school, I began to realize that my life was going nowhere. I was plagued with doubts about my future and suddenly faced with the reality of repeating the tenth grade for the third time. Also, my younger brother, began to follow in my footsteps. I didn't want him to live the life I had been living thus far. I also felt that I was a disappointment to my family. After all, my mother had worked so hard to support me. I also felt that I was a disappointment to my girlfriend, who excelled in school. She told me that she didn't want to go out with a "loser." I thought about the disappointment that I had caused my mother and my girlfriend. I also thought about what a bad example I was setting for my brother and sister. And finally, I began to think about what a disappointment I was to myself. So, I made a decision to change my life. I began to stay out of trouble and to attend school on a regular basis. However, I managed to get into a minor scrape within a short time after my commitment to stay on track. I was charged with violating probation for shooting a BB gun out my bedroom window.

I probably could have had the charges dismissed, but I didn't want them to be. This is because my probation officer told me about Ocean Tides School. Ocean Tides would allow me to make up all the schoolwork I had missed while giving me the structure in my life that I so badly needed. I decided that this was the way to go.

Since attending Ocean Tides School, I have turned my life around. I entered the Ocean Tides program on May 23, 1997. I only had four credits toward a high school diploma. I needed fourteen more credits in order to graduate. Through my commitment to turn my life around, I began to make up work that I missed. I have taken Double Credits English, Spanish, and attended summer school. Through hard work and perseverance, I began to meet my goals. I have received straight A's since entering Ocean Tides. More importantly, is the fact that I now feel good about myself and no longer have the desire to fail. I now want only to succeed.

I plan on graduating from Ocean Tides High School this spring. I will be the first member of my family to graduate from high school. I will also be the first (family's last name) to ever attend college. Currently, I am enrolled in the Preparatory Enrollment Program (PEP) at Rhode Island College. This program is designed to prepare me for my full entrance into RIC. I attended PEP this spring and will continue throughout the summer.

I will be a full-time student at Rhode Island College in the fall. I am considering majoring in Counseling and Psychology. I hope with my degree and my life experiences that I can work with troubled youth some day. I believe that the Terence M. Handrigan Memorial Scholarship will help me continue my studies at RIC, as well has helping me to stay on the positive course I have chosen.

CONCLUSIONS

It would be difficult to judge any of these cases either as strictly success stories or failures because these boys' lives are too complex for that kind of assessment. Rather, their young lives are stories of resilience in the face of adversity and almost insurmountable hardship—intermittent successes mingled with disappointments and struggles, the likes of which most young boys growing up in America never have to encounter. The Ocean Tides program was there for these boys providing care, guidance, counseling, and family support systems in the role of surrogate parents sometimes for more than a year of their young lives, and other times forging relationships with these young men that would last a lifetime.

CHAPTER 10

Sailing Home: Final Thoughts

Rehabilitating male juvenile delinquents is a difficult, multifaceted, and trying process fraught with political, budgetary, and attitudinal problems and obstacles. Since the term *juvenile delinquency* was coined in the 1700s, people have been struggling to find ways to address this social problem. Our research indicates that one successful way to attend to it is to employ a positive approach to rehabilitation based on relationship building and providing essential skills that can lead to significant changes in behavior. In this book, we have described an innovative residential and treatment program and provided useful empirical information gathered from a painstakingly detailed examination of the lives of a large group of young male juvenile delinquents. This information can be used to inform people working in rehabilitation programs with delinquents, politicians and others responsible for establishing policy, and academicians who teach about juvenile delinquency. The research study, which is the largest of its kind to gather data from multiple sources, is a valuable source of information about the causes of delinquency and key issues in rehabilitating adolescent male juvenile delinquents.

The young men described in this book are not like other boys their age. They are more likely to be poor, deficient in basic educational and social skills, and lacking positive family and social support networks. Contrary to the popular beliefs, they are not inherently bad or evil, but are missing some of the essential elements necessary for success in life. Instead of thinking of them as broken, it is more adaptive to conceptualize them as incomplete. The task of rehabilitation is to make them whole by filling in the structural and emotional voids they need to function better in society on into adulthood.

Instead of focusing on what is wrong with the juvenile justice system and how to fix it, which has been characteristic of many studies on juvenile delinquency, we have examined the lives of juvenile offenders prior to entering the juvenile justice system in order to find its causes and to inform rehabilitation and prevention. One of the main theoretical bases for the manuscript is Robert Agnew's general theory of crime for explaining why some boys deviate from normative society.

AGNEW'S GENERAL STRAIN THEORY AND CAUSATION

Based on decades of empirical evidence from research and explanations for crime and delinquency from multiple theories that identify the experiences that lead to crime, Agnew's theory explains that crime is a way of coping with strains that come from cultural, social, and individual experiences. These strains cause an imbalance of reinforcements over constraints against criminal coping. For the boys in this study who have already engaged in criminal activities, Agnew's theory provides useful guidelines for rehabilitation.

In Agnew's theory, the family is the most important of the life domains. Family is a key ingredient in the development of the self. Although the family's influence diminishes as the child grows into adolescence and peer pressure challenges parental guidance for priority, an examination of childhood experiences is a good place to look for the potential causes of delinquent behavior that may not show up until later. Our research results show that exposure to a bad family environment, particularly witnessing or experiencing parental interpersonal violence, has devastating effects on children, but those ill effects can be diminished with the right interventions. Boys exposed to violence in their homes are much more likely to become violent against others. Removing them from their home and putting them in an environment where bad parenting is replaced by positive parental role models has a beneficial effect, particularly on diminishing their violent behavior.

THE OCEAN TIDES EFFECT

Although many people are in favor of keeping troubled youngsters with their families and treating them as outpatients in their local communities, residential placement is necessary when a youngster becomes unmanageable at home or community-based interventions have failed. Unfortunately, many adjudicated boys are sent to youth prisons, also commonly known as "reform schools" or "training schools," which are predominantly punitive, ignore their families, and do not prepare boys for reintegration into the community and their homes once they have served their sentences. Despite the predominance of these custodial programs, there is little or no evidence to show that these programs offer effective treatment or models for improved social functioning. It is much more effective to work directly with the families and the delinquent youth in a structured but supportive environment for an extended period of time than it is to simply punish them and release them back into the community.

The Ocean Tides program is a residential program that is an alternative to youth prison. It is a structured program that includes individualized education in an excellent school, individual and family counseling for every resident, closely supervised residential life, and a variety of recreational activities for the residents. The program has a number of special activities designed to help the residents develop necessary personal and social skills, provide them with new experiences, and expand their awareness of the world outside of their limited environmental backgrounds. The program is designed to reduce unnecessary strain, provide the young men with positive alternatives to criminal activities, and help raise their levels of self-esteem. Two key components of the program are the provision of regular family counseling while the young men are in residence and gradually transitioning them back into the community by placing them in smaller group homes where they learn how to cook, clean, and care for themselves. Recently, there has been an emphasis on positive youth development that is influencing how rehabilitation programs are structured and administered. Ocean Tides was ahead of its time and has used this model since its inception in 1975. Our research indicates that this is a move in the right direction.

THE IMPORTANCE OF CLINICAL CONSULTANTS

A major problem in dealing with juvenile delinquents in residential programs is staff burnout and turnover. Dealing with these kids can be emotionally taxing and difficult in practice. For a program to be successful, constant self-examination, development of new ideas and new approaches, ongoing training and attention to the emotional welfare of the staff, and regular evaluations of staff job performance are required. One of the ways of accomplishing these goals is through the use of outside consultants to provide in-service training, monitor and mediate staff conflicts, facilitate the discussion and brainstorming of new ideas, and provide expertise in the delivery of special services. We have described how Ocean Tides uses both outside consultants with special expertise and a regular consultant in clinical psychology to maintain the program at a high level of functioning.

One of the important functions of the consultant in clinical psychology is to do an assessment of referred residents that describes their psychological profile and identifies positive attributes that can be used as a basis for designing and implementing an individual treatment plan for their rehabilitation. Although interviewing these young men can be difficult because of their mistrust of adult authority figures in general and mental health professionals in particular, the curiosity model of interviewing that is explained in this book increases the chances of establishing a relationship with the boys and obtaining useful information that is important to rehabilitation.

WHAT HAS HAPPENED SINCE 2007?

In assessing what has happened to the program since the completion of the data collection in 2007, the phrase "all good things must come to an end" unfortunately comes to mind. Despite the success of the program and the continued support of the family court judges in Rhode Island, the program has experienced a significant downsizing due in part to budget cuts from the state and the Department of Children, Youth and Families, which are the primary sources of funding for the program, and in part as the result of changes in the state's system of coordinating placements. The relevant social services agencies within the state have been organized into two networks that are responsible for managing placements. Although the family court judges continue to have discretion over the placement of adjudicated boys in Rhode Island, their recommendations are not always followed or are not implemented in a timely manner by the networks.

The size of Ocean Tides has been reduced from 65 available beds to 35 beds. Most of this reduction has occurred from the gradual closing of all four of the community-based extension houses or group homes. The first house was closed in 2008, followed by a second closing in 2011 and the final two closings occurring in 2013. The closing of these facilities has seriously damaged the ability of the program to maintain a community presence. It has also removed the opportunity to gradually transition the boys' return to their homes or the community by allowing them to live in a smaller and more intimate environment where they can develop essential life skills. Now 18-year-old boys who often have few or no social support networks are being told to make it on their own in an economic and social climate in which most 20-somethings are still in their parents' homes even after completing college. This unrealistic expectation significantly increases recidivism and undermines the work that is being done at Ocean Tides.

A change in the state's reimbursement policy has also seriously affected Ocean Tides. Prior to 2006, if Ocean Tides kept 90% of its beds filled, it received 100% of its allotment for the year. In 2008, the system of reimbursement changed to a per diem so that any day that a bed is not filled, the program is not paid. In a residential program, temporary vacant beds are inevitable due to residents completing the program, runaways, and some residents being returned to the training school because of noncompliance. The change in reimbursement placed severe and ultimately unmanageable financial hardships on the program.

The length of time boys are sentenced to Ocean Tides has also been significantly reduced. The Ocean Tides program was designed to be 1 year in length because this was the minimal amount of time deemed necessary to accomplish the goals of treatment. With these young men it takes time to establish a relationship and for them to accept the structure and limits of the program. With recent and current sentences as short as 3 months, this does not provide enough time to accomplish what the program is designed to do. Our research clearly shows the effectiveness of a program that is based on 1 year in residence. There is no indication that a shorter program will be as effective in rehabilitating youthful offenders. Two additional indications of the importance of continuity to the success of the program are the stability of the staff and the rewards they experience from developing close relationships with the residents. There has been amazingly little turnover among staff despite limited salaries, and many former residents return to visit after completing the program and/or maintain contact with various staff members and administrators on into their adulthood.

A more general trend away from residential placement for adjudicated boys has precipitated some of these decisions. In part, this trend is a reaction to the overcrowding that occurred in youth prisons in the 1980s and 1990s. The nationally high rate of recidivism for boys who have been sentenced to youth prisons is another reason for the trend toward keeping them home. However, the policy overgeneralizes residential programs as one of two types—the youth prison or nondelinquent child welfare placements.

Another contributing factor to the trend away from placing youngsters in residential programs is a belief that children are better off with their own parents. There are some youngsters who, by virtue of the seriousness of their crimes or their behavior in other ways, have to be removed from the home. This is necessary for both the welfare of the youngster and the welfare of the family. Removal from the home does not necessarily mean that the family is being neglected. On the contrary, Ocean Tides has an active program of family counseling that is maintained throughout the duration of the boys' stay in the program. Most of this family work occurs either in home visits or a location convenient to the family. The closing of the various group homes eliminated a number of locations around the state that were close to where the families lived and provided convenient places in which the family counseling sessions could take place.

These are all unfortunate developments from both a financial and treatment efficacy perspective. These changes increase juvenile recidivism, and significantly decrease rehabilitation strategies that result in increased crime and unemployment, substantial burden on the entire criminal justice system, and decreases in job satisfaction and security for those who are employed to help these youngsters. Financially, it is clear that a training school or youth prison is the most expensive facility in which to place a juvenile. In Rhode Island, the cost of placing a youngster at Ocean Tides in 2013 is 63% less than that of keeping him in the training school. If limits in state revenue are driving budget cuts and there is a necessity to save money by reducing expenses, it makes no sense to reduce the least expensive and most effective programs in favor of the most expensive and least effective. From a treatment perspective, there is no evidence that placing a youngster in a youth prison does anything positive to help his rehabilitation or teach him new skills. On the contrary, it appears that the only new skills the young men acquire are new and better ways to commit crime. They do not establish the positive relationships or get the kind of effective surrogate parenting, family and individual counseling, and educational opportunities that they get in programs like Ocean Tides. Likewise, returning a boy to his dysfunctional family prematurely is paramount to doing nothing at all.

WHERE DO WE GO FROM HERE? IMPLICATIONS FOR PUBLIC POLICY

There is an old saying: "There is no arguing with a closed mind." Unfortunately, juvenile crime and the perception of those who commit it frequently stimulate a "closed mind"–response not only from the general public, but from the public officials who establish policy and determine the nature of rehabilitation efforts. For many people, fear of crime is associated with the political aphorism "get tough on crime." Even among knowledgeable experts, stereotyping, overgeneralization, and prejudice exist. For example, in submitting grant applications to support the research reported in this book, it was clear that many reviewers felt that these boys were a lost cause. Your local and national politicians are aware of the prejudices and the fear that generate these kinds of responses and getting tougher on crime earns constituent support. However, it is shortsighted and decreases public security. When a politician says that he or she is going to "get tough on crime," it is important to ask why and to request that they provide not only a logical rationale, but evidence to support that approach.

In order to obtain the necessary evidence, there is a need for additional research that is multidisciplinary, longitudinal, and in depth. Many of the previous findings about juvenile delinquency are based on data derived only from police records, phone interviews with delinquents, or other limited sources that cannot possibly tell us what we need to know. Empirically, sound research takes more time and more money to complete, but such investment is necessary to create positive structural changes in the criminal justice system that will improve security, corrections, education, family functioning, and the overall quality of life in American society. It just makes good sense to invest more time, resources, and positive strategies to make improvements in these young lives.

APPENDIX A

Additional Tables

TABLE A.1
Reason for Release From the Ocean Tides Program

REASON	*n*	PERCENT	VALID PERCENT
Unauthorized	207	13.1	13.4
Graduation	991	62.5	64.2
Returned to RITS	282	17.8	18.3
Terminated	64	4.0	4.1
Total	1,544	97.4	100
System missing	41	2.6	

Note: "Valid percent" is the percent of boys in each category out of the entire database, including those for whom we do not have this information, while "percent" is the percent of boys in each category only for whom we had this information.

RITS, Rhode Island Training School.

TABLE A.2
Socioeconomic Status (SES)

SES	*n*	PERCENT	VALID PERCENT
Underclass	402	25.4	26.9
Poverty	243	15.3	16.3
Lower middle	472	29.8	31.6
Middle range	333	21.0	22.3
Upper middle	42	2.6	2.8
Total	1,492	94.1	100
System missing	93	5.9	

Note: "Valid percent" is the percent of boys in each category out of the entire database, including those for whom we do not have this information, while "percent" is the percent of boys in each category only for whom we had this information.

TABLE A.3
Race and Ethnicity

RACE AND ETHNICITY	*n*	PERCENT	VALID PERCENT
Asian	37	2.3	2.8
Black	162	10.2	12.2
Cape Verdean	34	2.1	2.6
Hispanic White	47	3.0	3.6
Hispanic non-White	89	5.6	6.7
Hispanic nondescriptive	33	2.1	2.5
Puerto Rican	52	3.3	3.9
Native American	15	0.9	1.1
White	742	46.8	56.1
Multiracial	112	7.1	8.5
Total	1,323	83.5	100
System missing	262	16.5	

Note: "Valid percent" is the percent of boys in each category out of the entire database, including those for whom we do not have this information, while "percent" is the percent of boys in each category only for whom we had this information.

TABLE A.4
Race

RACE	*n*	PERCENT	VALID PERCENT
White	789	49.8	59.6
Non-White	534	33.7	40.4
Total	1,323	83.5	100
System missing	262	16.5	

Note: "Valid percent" is the percent of boys in each category out of the entire database, including those for whom we do not have this information, while "percent" is the percent of boys in each category only for whom we had this information.

TABLE A.5
Growth in Non-White OT Population Over Time

YEAR RANGE	# YEARS	# NON-WHITE	PERCENT OF TOTAL NON-WHITE
1975–1990	15	89	17
1991–1999	9	184	34
2000	1	50	9
2001–2006	6	211	40

OT, Ocean Tides.

TABLE A.6
Family Structure

FAMILY STRUCTURE	*n*	PERCENT	VALID PERCENT
More than one adult (total)	*812*	*52.2*	*51.2*
Both biological parents	390	24.6	25.1
Biological mother and stepfather	213	13.4	13.7
Biological mother and other father[a]	66	4.2	4.2
Biological father and stepmother	50	3.2	3.2
Biological mother and grandmother	40	2.5	2.6
Grandmother and grandfather	18	1.1	1.2
Biological father and grandmother	15	0.9	1.0
Biological father and other mother	11	0.7	0.7
Aunt and uncle	9	0.6	0.6
Single parent (total)	*707*	*45.5*	*44.6*
Biological mother only	545	34.4	35.1
Stepfather only	56	3.5	3.6
Other mother only	36	2.3	2.3
Grandmother only	29	1.8	1.9
A sibling only	13	0.8	0.8
Aunt only	12	0.8	0.8
Uncle only	7	0.4	0.5
Other father only	6	0.4	0.4
Stepmother only	2	0.1	0.1
Grandfather only	1	0.1	0.1
Unknown number of adults			
Foster care[b]	34	2.1	2.2

Note: Consistently throughout the database, "stepfather" and "stepmother" include only legally married couples because a 1-year rule for common law in Rhode Island does not exist as it does in many other states. "Valid percent" is the percent of boys in each category out of the entire database, including those for whom we do not have this information, while "percent" is the percent of boys in each category only for whom we had this information.

[a]For this variable, "other mother" and "other father" indicate some mother or father figure not otherwise listed here, such as a boyfriend or a girlfriend of a biological parent.

[b]In the state of Rhode Island, foster families can consist of single or multiple adults.

TABLE A.7
Family Stability

FAMILY STABILITY	*n*	PERCENT	VALID PERCENT
Stable	699	44.1	44.6
Moderately stable	585	36.9	37.3
Unstable	285	18.9	18.2
Total	1,569	99.0	100.0

Note: "Valid percent" is the percent of boys in each category out of the entire database, including those for whom we do not have this information, while "percent" is the percent of boys in each category only for whom we had this information.

TABLE A.8
Child Abuse

ABUSER	ABUSE			
	EMOTIONAL	PHYSICAL		SEXUAL
		No Serious Injury	Serious Injury	
Biological father	723 (45.6)	145 (9.1)	52 (3.3)	9 (0.6)
Stepfather	14 (0.9)	34 (2.1)	34 (2.1)	3 (0.2)
Other father	22 (1.4)	36 (2.3)	11 (0.7)	11 (0.7)
Biological mother	325 (20.5)	34 (2.1)	30 (1.9)	7 (0.4)
Stepmother	0	2 (0.1)	3 (0.2)	0
Other mother	4 (0.3)	4 (0.3)	1 (0.1)	2 (0.1)
Sibling	8 (0.5)	19 (1.2)	4 (0.3)	10 (0.6)
Other relative	5 (0.3)	8 (0.5)	4 (0.3)	25 (1.6)
Other nonrelative	5 (0.3)	42 (2.6)	29 (1.8)	54 (3.4)

Note: Percentage of Ocean Tides boys are given in parentheses. Some boys experienced multiple abuses from several family members.

TABLE A.9
Discipline at Home

DISCIPLINE	*n*	PERCENT	VALID PERCENT
None	196	12.4	17.4
Lenient	416	26.2	36.9
Moderate	258	16.3	22.9
Harsh	75	4.7	6.7
Inconsistent	181	11.4	16.1
Total	1,126	71.0	100
Missing	459	29.0	

Note: "Valid percent" is the percent of boys in each category out of the entire database, including those for whom we do not have this information, while "percent" is the percent of boys in each category only for whom we had this information.

TABLE A.10
Most Recent Charges

OFFICIAL CHARGE	*n*
Aggravated assault	136
Armed robbery	39
Arson	44
Attempted murder	13
Auto theft	207
Breaking and entering	444
Burglary	6
Credit-card fraud	20
Domestic assault	12
Driving with no license	122
Drug possession	132
Drug with intent to sell	113
Gun possession	119
Kidnapping	2
Malicious mischief	138
Murder	1
Prostitution	2
Resisting arrest	39
Robbery	134
Sexual assault (nonspecified)	32
Sexual assault—victim aged 0–15 years	19
Sexual assault—victim aged 16+ years	1
Simple assault	195
Theft	355
Trespassing	40
Vandalism	172
Violation of probation	506
Wayward (running away)	139
Total	3,182

Note: "Most recent charges" include multiple charges against single offenders.

TABLE A.11
Behavioral Medications

ANTIANXIETY		ANTIDEPRESSANT		ANTIPSYCHOTIC		STIMULANT	
Past	At OT	Past	At OT	Past	At OT	Past	At OT
24 (1.5)	6 (0.4)	99 (6.2)	42 (2.6)	8 (0.5)	4 (0.3)	192 (12.1)	5 (0.3)

Note: Percents in parentheses.
OT, Ocean Tides.

TABLE A.12
Past Behavioral Medications by SES

SES	ANTIANXIETY	ANTIDEPRESSANT	ANTIPSYCHOTIC	STIMULANT
Underclass and borderline poverty	6 (0.9%)	32 (5.0%)	1 (0.2%)	59 (9.1%)
Middle range	16 (2.0%)	59 (7.3%)	7 (0.9%)	114 (14.2%)
Upper middle	1 (2.4%)	5 (11.0%)	0	12 (28.6%)
Kendall's tau-b (standard error)	*.043 (.024)*	*.056 (.025)**	*.041 (.018)*	*.097 (.025)***

SES, socioeconomic status.
$n = 1{,}492$.
$^{*}p < .05$. $^{**}p < .000$.

TABLE A.13
Past School Performance Prior to Ocean Tides

SCHOOL PERFORMANCE	ACADEMICS	MOTIVATION	BEHAVIOR
Consistently poor	741 (46.8)	885 (55.8)	795 (50.2)
Consistently average	235 (14.8)	185 (11.7)	225 (14.2)
Consistently above average	60 (3.8)	33 (2.1)	40 (2.5)
Variable	176 (11.1)	126 (7.9)	127 (8)
Average poor to poor average	252 (15.9)	184 (11.6)	222 (14.0)
Totals	1,464 (92.4)	1,413 (89.1)	1,409 (88.9)
Missing	121 (7.6)	172 (10.9)	176 (11.1)

Note: Percents in parentheses.

TABLE A.14
Childhood Development

DEVELOPMENT	*n*	PERCENT	VALID PERCENT
Below average	118	7.4	9.0
Normal/average	1,174	74.1	89.1
Above average	25	1.6	1.9
Total	1,317	83.1	100
Missing	268	16.9	

Note: "Valid percent" is the percent of boys in each category out of the entire database, including those for whom we do not have this information, while "percent" is the percent of boys in each category only for whom we had this information.

TABLE A.15
Career Goals

CAREER GOALS	*n*	PERCENT
Armed forces	122	7.7
Carpenter/construction	99	6.2
Computer/technical	33	2.1
Drug dealer	6	0.4
Lawyer	18	1.1
Mechanic	88	5.6
Police officer	24	1.5
Professional sports	39	2.5
Work with kids	11	0.7
Teacher	13	0.8
Just to have a job	4	0.3
Truck driver	8	0.5
Trades—electrician, plumber, etc.	26	1.6
Cook	25	1.6
Sales/business	13	0.8
Commercial fishing	9	0.6
Commercial arts	18	1.1
Medicine	19	1.2
Entertainment industry	14	0.9

TABLE A.16
Hobbies

HOBBIES	*n*	PERCENT
Art	193	12.2
College	181	11.4
Hanging out with friends	193	12.2
Motorcycles/dirt bikes/4 wheeling	89	5.6
Playing music	84	5.3
Listening to music	101	6.4
Reading	68	4.3
Sports	881	55.6
Trouble	38	2.4
Watching TV	67	4.2
Writing	20	1.3
Outdoor activities	54	3.4
Cards/board games	22	1.4
Cooking	28	1.8
Mechanics	40	2.5
Fitness/dance	21	1.3
Video games	29	1.8
Computers	19	1.2

APPENDIX B

Administrator Performance Evaluation Form: Ocean Tides, Inc.

Name of Administrator: ________________ Title: ________________
Department: ________________ Date of Evaluation: ________________
Rating Period: / / to / /

Instructions: Carefully evaluate and rate each of the performance characteristics listed below based on recurring day-to-day performance and not on recent or isolated, exceptional events. For each characteristic, rate the administrator as poor, fair, average, good, or excellent using the rating definitions listed as follows and check the appropriate space. Comments may be written in the space below each factor. This form should be completed anonymously to ensure candid evaluation.

Excellent (**Exc.**): Outstanding; unquestionably above acceptable standards; performance consistently exceeds job requirements.

Good: Above acceptable standards; performance usually exceeds job requirements.

Average (Avr.): Meets acceptable standards; performance of job requirements is consistent.

Fair: Improvement is needed to meet acceptable standards; performance of job requirements is inconsistent.

Poor: Definitely below acceptable standards; performance of job requirements is consistent deficient.

Poor	Fair	Avr.	Good	Exc.	
___	___	___	___	___	1. **JOB KNOWLEDGE:** Understands skills, methods, and procedures required in position and is able to perform required duties.
___	___	___	___	___	2. **PLANNING:** Development of methods to efficiently perform overall workload.
___	___	___	___	___	3. **APPLICATION:** Ensures consistent job performance to complete overall workload.
___	___	___	___	___	4. **THOROUGHNESS:** Attention to requisite details of job; completes tasks.
___	___	___	___	___	5. **QUALITY**: Accuracy and thoroughness of work.
___	___	___	___	___	6. **PRODUCTIVITY:** Quantity or volume of work done under normal conditions.
___	___	___	___	___	7. **RELIABILITY/DEPENDABILITY:** Observes work schedule; meets deadlines; adheres to policies.
___	___	___	___	___	8. **ATTITUDE/COOPERATION:** Interest in job; effectiveness in working with others.
___	___	___	___	___	9. **SUPERVISORY SKILLS:** Effectiveness as a supervisor; provides guidance and helpful feedback.
___	___	___	___	___	10. **MANAGEMENT OF RESIDENTS:** Skilled in dealing with residents; ability to set limits and sanction appropriately and to provide support and positive feedback.
___	___	___	___	___	11. **LEADERSHIP:** Models effective job performance; takes charge and inspires staff to do their best; supports and encourages staff.
___	___	___	___	___	12. **COMMUNICATION SKILLS:** Effective presentation of information in written

and verbal forms; clear direct and honest in communication with staff and residents.

____ ____ ____ ____ ____ 13. **ADMINISTRATIVE SKILLS:** Ability to organize and structure work; attentive to necessary details; effective problem solver.

____ ____ ____ ____ ____ 14. **WORK HABITS:** Conscientious and diligent in carrying out responsibilities; completes tasks in timely fashion.

____ ____ ____ ____ ____ 15. **JUDGMENT:** Ability to apply common sense and make good decisions by careful study of available information and options.

____ ____ ____ ____ ____ 16. **INTERPERSONAL RELATIONS:** Ability to work comfortably and effectively with staff and residents; shows empathy, support, and understanding.

____ ____ ____ ____ ____ 17. **CREATIVITY:** Uses imaginative and innovative thinking in carrying out responsibilities; develops new ideas.

____ ____ ____ ____ ____ 18. **INITIATIVE**: Self-confident, enthusiastic performance of tasks.

____ ____ ____ ____ ____ 19. **ECONOMY:** Proper and prudent use of facilities, equipment, and materials; good management of resources.

____ ____ ____ ____ ____ 20. **PERSEVERANCE**: Able to perform duties in face of frustration, opposition, or discouragement.

COMMENTS:

MAJOR STRENGTHS:

MAJOR WEAKNESSES:

SUGGESTIONS/RECOMMENDATIONS:

APPENDIX C

Sample Reports

TWO EXAMPLES OF INTERVIEWS WITH GUARDED RESIDENTS

Clinical Psychological Evaluation

Name: Haroldo (*Note:* Names have been changed.)

Referral: Haroldo is a recently readmitted resident at the Narragansett Campus of Ocean Tides. Haroldo originally came to Ocean Tides in [month/year]. He went AWOL after 4 days and was readmitted to the program on [month/year] after being in the Youth Detention Center at the training school for 5 months. Haroldo was referred for a clinical psychological evaluation.

Behavioral observations: Haroldo is a 15-year-old, light-complexioned young man of mixed Cape Verdean and Portuguese ethnicity. He is of average height with a thin, wiry build. Haroldo has closely cut dark brown hair and no facial hair. He was not wearing any earrings or other jewelry and has no visible scars, tattoos, or other distinguishing marks. He accompanied me with some hesitation. Before I could explain the purpose of our contact, he inquired as to my identity and "what this was all about." Haroldo maintained this cautious and guarded attitude throughout the interview. He was cordial, but distant and wary. Haroldo answered questions carefully and with minimal information, often pausing before he responded. He did not volunteer any information but answered follow-up questions. His mood was serious and bordered on sullen. He smiled on a couple of occasions. Haroldo sat still and maintained eye contact. He did not express any unusual ideas or exhibit any behavior that was out of the ordinary. The evaluation was completed successfully but with difficulty.

Interview

Family: Haroldo lives in South Providence with his mother and 19-year-old sister. Haroldo is the youngest of six children, three males and three females. All of the other siblings live outside of the home. He did not know the ages of his older siblings, but said that the oldest is 25 years old. Two of his sisters have children (two each). His mother does not work and he said that she spends a lot of time watching television. When I asked him if she drank alcohol, he responded: "once in a while." Haroldo reported that she used to work at Wal-Mart. He described his mother as "a very good cook" and said that they get along well. Haroldo did not provide much information about his father. He said that he has not seen his father in about a year. His father lives in the Fox Point section of Providence. Haroldo could not provide any additional information about his father.

Charges: Haroldo is in custody for breaking and entering. He committed the crime with two friends. They were apprehended hiding behind a garage. Unlike most residents, he did not provide much information about his charge. He stated that this was his first attempt at breaking and entering. He revealed one prior charge of arson when he was 13 years old. Haroldo stated that he lit the corner of a piece of construction paper on fire and immediately put it out. He maintained that the paper did not even catch on fire before he extinguished it. Despite this, he was charged with arson and placed on probation.

Substance use: Haroldo admitted to heavy and regular use of marijuana prior to being incarcerated. He reported that he would smoke five or six blunts a day and admitted to selling marijuana occasionally. Haroldo smokes five or six cigarettes a day and stated that he misses the cigarettes more than the pot. He used to drink alcohol but no longer does. Haroldo denied use of any other drugs.

Interests, plans for the future, and prior school adjustment: Haroldo was attending the V School "for behavior problems" prior to coming to Ocean Tides. He has few interests or hobbies other than hanging out with his friends and family. He indicated that he plays sports at Ocean Tides, but does not play when he is on his own. Haroldo has a girlfriend and reported that she is currently on home confinement for stealing a cell phone. Haroldo would like to finish high school. His career plans are indefinite. He thought about going into real estate but several people have told him that he could lose a lot of money, so he is rethinking that idea.

Impressions

Haroldo is an extremely guarded and self-contained young man, who, by his own admission, has "an edge." He was very careful about the information he gave and it was my impression that he was telling me what he thought I wanted to hear rather than being candid and truthful. Haroldo has a considerable amount of internalized and unexpressed anger. Haroldo acknowledged that when people get on his nerves, he "feels like slapping (in distinction to hitting) them" but does not do it. While he had trouble finding the exact words to label his moods, Haroldo described being irritable much of the time. He stated that these moods come on him randomly and with no obvious environmental trigger or provocation. Haroldo reported that his mother has told him that he "does not like anybody and is mad at the world." Haroldo does not disagree with her assessment. Although Haroldo is able to describe his moods, he has no insight or awareness of why they occur. He admitted that people, particularly adults (in distinction to peers), get on his nerves easily and he does not like being told what to do. It was clear that Haroldo was carefully censoring the information he reported and there were some obvious contradictions. For example, he told me that he likes to spend his free time hanging out with his family but could not tell me how old his siblings were.

Haroldo presents with the classic adolescent pattern of depression, in which irritability replaces dysphoria as the predominant symptom. Although Haroldo did not report any current symptoms of depression, such as sadness, low energy, or eating and sleeping difficulties, he looks and sounds depressed. Haroldo said that he used to have trouble sleeping and was on sleep medication, but is sleeping fine now. He also eats well while at Ocean Tides. However, he says that he has little appetite when he goes home, even though his mother is a good cook. Haroldo attributes his loss of appetite to smoking cigarettes when at home. He did not report any past, recent, or current suicidal ideas or attempts.

Despite his internalized anger and his admission that there are some staff members he "would like to slap," I do not think Haroldo is at risk to harm staff or others by expressing his anger physically.

Haroldo explained that he ran away from the program initially because he did not like it but stated that he likes it better now after spending time at the training school. His adjustment to the program since returning has been marginal. He admitted to losing a couple of weekends for "stupid stuff," such as having sagging pants when he was on the Washington trip. However, he does not admit to being at fault but attributes the cause to a difference of opinion about clothing style. In this particular case, he indicated that Br. Brendan (who gave the sanction) wears his pants "way up here," pointing to his waist. Haroldo's perception is that whenever he is disciplined, others are treating him unfairly. For example, he expressed annoyance at being "thrown out of the anger management group" because he had to go to the bathroom. He was critical of the leader of the anger management group because "she talks down to you and she's got an attitude." As the aforementioned examples suggest, externalizing and projecting blame are two of Haroldo's main methods of coping with problems.

DSM-IV Diagnosis:

312.82 Conduct Disorder, Adolescent-Onset

305.20 Cannabis Abuse (in remission by virtue of incarceration)

300.4 Dysthymic Disorder With Atypical Features (R/O)

Recommendations

Although Haroldo stated that he likes Ocean Tides better the second time around, I question how seriously he is taking the program and how invested he is in changing his behavior. He acknowledges that he does not like talking to counselors about his problems. Haroldo stated that he likes to keep things in and work them out by himself. Even though he needs and could benefit from the present treatment plan that includes individual counseling, anger management, and drug counseling, he is likely to resist these treatment options by passive-aggressive behaviors, such as silence and noncompliance. Unless there is a major change in his present attitude, he will go through the motions of minimal external compliance with the demands of the program with little internalization of the goals and values of the program. If his frustration level builds, he may go AWOL again. Based on my current assessment, I think the prognosis for successful rehabilitation is minimal.

Clinical Psychological Evaluation

Name: Kevin

Referral: Kevin is a resident at the Narragansett Campus of Ocean Tides. He was referred for a clinical psychological evaluation after an episode yesterday during which he became very upset and threatened to go AWOL. The teachers were concerned about Kevin and recommended that he be seen for an evaluation.

Behavioral observations: Kevin is a tall, thin, 17-year-old African American young man with short hair. He was cleanly groomed and neatly dressed in the school uniform. Kevin was not wearing any earrings or other jewelry. He has a tattoo on each forehand. On his right hand is the word "Big" in Old English script and the word "Guy" in similar letters is on his left hand. Kevin said that this represented the nickname that was given to him by his mother at birth. He reported that these are the only tattoos that he has. Kevin does not have any visible scars or other distinguishing marks. Kevin accompanied me willingly and was pleasant, cordial, and cooperative. His demeanor was extremely "laid back." He talked and moved slowly and slouched in his chair, resting his head against the back of the chair. His posture seemed representative of the image he wants to present to others, which is languid, lackadaisical, nonchalant, and "cool." Kevin answered questions with some hesitation and his initial responses provided only the essential information. Consequently, I had to ask a number of follow-up questions to get detailed and more informative responses. Kevin exhibited a good sense of humor and laughed at times. Although he was a challenge to interview, the evaluation was completed successfully.

Interview

Family: Kevin lives with his maternal aunt and grandmother in Providence. The grandmother lives in an elderly apartment building. Kevin's aunt has been staying with her, although she is supposed to be looking for her own apartment. Kevin moved to Rhode Island about 6 years ago from Brooklyn, New York, where his mother and father reside. His mother and aunt are twin sisters. When I told him that I had heard that his mother had sent him to live with his aunt to keep him out of trouble, he corrected me and said that it was his father who had sent him. Kevin reported that he had not been in any trouble with the law in New York, but had not been going to school. His father works for the sanitation department. Kevin referred to him as a "garbage man." His parents were never married and have four children together. Each of them has five additional children with other partners (four other women for his father and a comparable number of men for his mother) so that between them they have sired 14 children. I asked Kevin in what way his mother and aunt were alike and he said, "They both lie." Kevin has a very conflicted relationship with his aunt. He said that she wants him back in the training school or at the Rhode Island Adult Correctional Institute. Kevin said that they used to get along but have had a falling out. He described an incident in which he wanted to go visit his infant son who resides with his former girlfriend. His aunt, who does not like his former girlfriend, did not want him to go. Kevin went anyway and stayed out all night. In addition to being a liar, Kevin described his aunt as an emotionally erratic woman whom other people refer to as "bipolar." He said that she used to have a shop where she sold clothes and cut hair in the back, but she closed the shop. Kevin said that his father had been sending his aunt money to cover Kevin's share of the rent, but he told his father to stop sending money.

Charges: Kevin stated that he did not begin getting into trouble with the law until he moved to Rhode Island. He is in custody for a robbery and assault charge. Kevin reported that he did not do the robbery, but "took the rap" for someone else. The assault charge came as a result of a "brawl" that occurred outside of high school. Kevin reported that someone "jumped" one of his friends and Kevin intervened in his friend's behalf. Suddenly, a melee involving "twenty or thirty" people resulted and Kevin said that he "took the rap." Kevin stated that he has no prior charges but indicated that he has committed a number of break-ins and personal robberies.

Substance use: Kevin admitted to occasional use of marijuana. He reported that he usually smokes when he gets drunk. Kevin prefers alcohol to pot and drinks mostly on weekends. He denied use of any other drugs.

Interests, plans for the future, and prior school adjustment: Kevin has a poor track record in school. He candidly admitted that he was expelled from several junior high schools, including R W, Greg S, and N. He finally completed E H Middle School. He was attending M P High School but was also expelled from there. His expulsions were usually for fighting but also for not doing the work. Kevin stated that he does not particularly like school but wants to go to college. He has no idea why he wants to go to college or even if he could "get through it." His interests are sports, particularly basketball. He was planning on trying out for the M P team and thinks he would have made it, but he was expelled prior to tryouts. Kevin said that his grades were never good enough to be eligible for the junior high teams. He likes to go to clubs, but was vague and evasive about any other interests. Kevin has no idea of what he wants to do to earn a living. He stated that most jobs that he could get would not pay as well as what he could make from stealing.

Impressions

Kevin is sort of an enigma. He is a pleasant young man that teachers and other staff describe as cooperative and a positive influence on other residents by intervening in conflicts and helping to break up fights. He was refreshingly candid in the interview, but many of his comments suggested that he is comfortable with his criminal activities. In some ways, Kevin is a throwback to some of the earlier residents of the program whose charges consisted primarily of breaking, entering, and robbery. Like them, Kevin spoke openly of his breaking into houses and stealing from individuals. He spoke in detail about how stealing a cell phone is the easiest and most lucrative way to rob someone. Kevin described how he can just walk by and grab the phone out of a person's hand. He shared his knowledge about the street value of different phones depending on whether a phone plan was needed to use them. This was the only topic in the interview that he talked about easily and in detail. Kevin said that he has never been caught stealing and implied an attitude of invulnerability in the sense that he does not think he would be caught. He revealed that he keeps about half of the items he steals for himself and the rest he sells.

Kevin impressed me as headstrong, opinionated, and fatalistic. He expressed the belief that the time of one's death is determined at birth and when your time comes, there is nothing you can do to prevent it. This was in the context of discussing that he has been shot at but never hit. In talking about his 1-year-old son, Kevin commented that the baby cries a lot and is spoiled. Kevin thinks that the child's mother spoils him and that he is the only one who disciplines him. When I asked him how he does it, Kevin said he would "hit him" and explained that he would lightly tap the child's hand. He admitted that he would hit the child when he was older if it was necessary. When I pointed out that hitting a child to discipline him is now considered child abuse and is not acceptable, he rejected this idea, adding, "The problem with half the kids in here is that they were never disciplined." With regard to his wanting to go AWOL, he said the main reason he did not leave was because the staff would not give him his cell phone. He stated that he had paid a lot of money for the phone and was not going to leave without it.

Kevin did not express any remorse or guilt for his past actions. On the contrary, he seems to be comfortable with and committed to making money the easiest way possible. He does not appear at this time to be motivated to do what is necessary to learn a legitimate occupation. Kevin acknowledged that he does not plan ahead or think about the future and that most of his actions are spontaneous. This was clear from his responses. For example, Kevin seemed unaware of the discrepancy between his past school performance and his desire to go to college. His main reason for wanting to graduate from college is to make his grandmother proud of him. Kevin is upset about the present situation with his aunt, but he is not clinically depressed and does not show any signs of a thought disorder or any other psychological disorder.

DSM-IV Diagnosis:

312.82 Conduct Disorder, Adolescent-Onset Type

Recommendations

The main challenge with this young man will be to try and get him to internalize some of the values of the program and develop the motivation to alter his current lifestyle. Individual counseling should focus on helping him evaluate some of the choices he is making. He could also benefit from some training on how to be a more effective parent. Kevin does not need any other special programming.

EXAMPLE OF AN INTERVIEW WITH A PARTIALLY RESPONSIVE RESIDENT

Clinical Psychological Evaluation

Name: Carlos

Referral: Carlos is a recently readmitted resident at the Narragansett Campus of Ocean Tides. He was referred for a clinical psychological evaluation.

Behavioral observations: Carlos is a tall, lean, 17-year-old young man of Puerto Rican ethnicity. He has closely cut brown hair and a carefully trimmed mustache and beard. Although we had never talked before, Carlos had seen me around at the Providence Campus, so he knew who I was. He was pleasant and friendly on introduction and shook hands. Carlos accompanied me willingly. He was polite, respectful, and cooperative during the interview. His mood was upbeat and he smiled frequently. Carlos showed some restlessness by moving around in his chair, but he maintained eye contact throughout the interview. His responses to questions varied considerably. He answered some questions with a reasonable degree of completeness and added additional information spontaneously. At other times, he appeared uncomfortable revealing information and would laugh. Carlos paused before answering certain questions and appeared to be censoring his response. However, he appeared to be candid and sincere and the information he reported is consistent with the information in his file. Carlos did not exhibit any unusual behavior or express any ideas that were out of the ordinary. The evaluation was completed successfully.

Interview

Family: Carlos lives in Newport with his mother, stepfather, and two younger brothers, aged 14 and 15 years. His mother and biological father divorced when he was 6 years old. Carlos described his father as an alcoholic and drug abuser, who used to beat his mother. Carlos witnessed the abuse. I asked him if his father was drunk or sober when he would hit his mother. Carlos replied: "I was only six and didn't know if he was drunk or sober." Occasionally, his father would hit the children. Carlos reported that his mother started dating her current husband about a year after the divorce but they did not marry until 4 years ago. His mother works as a manager of a Wendy's restaurant. His stepfather was formerly the manager of the same restaurant but now works in road construction for the X Corporation. Carlos reported contradictory information about his relationship with his parents. Initially, he stated that he gets along well with them but then added that he has a history of conflict and arguments with his mother. Carlos reported that she would set limits on his behavior by not letting him go out or disciplining him for not keeping his curfew. He said: "I have a very bad temper" and admitted that at times he would hit his mother when he was younger. Carlos mentioned that one of his younger brothers is doing well but the other one recently completed 2 years on probation for taking a knife to school. Carlos has not had any contact with his father for several years. He used to see him occasionally. Carlos said that his father is somewhere in Connecticut. He said that he is disabled from a back injury and used to work in construction. As far as he knows, his father still drinks.

Charges: Carlos was in the final stages of completing the Ocean Tides program when he picked up new charges of felony assault. He reported that he hit another kid with a metal baseball bat. Carlos said that he hit him twice, once in the chest and once in the head. He described the incident as follows. Carlos was at some girl's house where he was going to fight her boyfriend. She was hitting and slapping Carlos and trying to push him off the steps of the porch. The victim, whom he described as "a big guy that was drunk," came after Carlos. The bat was lying around and apparently they both went for it and Carlos got it first. Carlos reported that this is his fourth charge assault. Two of his prior charges were simple assaults for being involved in fights. The other one was also a felony assault charge also involving the use of a baseball bat.

Substance use: Carlos admitted to prior regular use of marijuana. He has also used Ecstasy at parties but denied use of any other drugs. Carlos said that when he smoked marijuana, he used a lot. When I asked where he got the money for the pot, Carlos explained that he had friends who gave it to him. He also reluctantly admitted to selling marijuana but indicated that he has never been apprehended or charged. In talking about his drug use, Carlos was very cautious.

Interests, plans for the future, and prior school adjustment: Carlos is in the 11th grade but acknowledged that he has a history of doing poorly in school. For example, he likes sports, particularly baseball and basketball, and would have liked to play on a high school team but his grades were not good enough. Carlos also indicated that he used to like to box when he was younger, but never participated in an organized program. Carlos attributes his poor performance in school to an inability to concentrate because of too many distractions, particularly "girls." He has done better at the Ocean Tides School because of the smaller classes and not having the distraction of girls being in the classes. A recent (May, 2009) psychological/neuropsychological evaluation indicated that both his overall IQ and Verbal Comprehension were in the Borderline Range (FSIQ of 79). His thinking and reasoning skills exceed only 8% of his peers. These limited cognitive skills would contribute significantly to his difficulties in learning and in school. His career goals are to finish high school, hopefully next year, and to get a job in construction. Carlos is hoping that his stepfather can get him a job with Carlos Construction. He mentioned that his stepfather's father worked for Carlos and that is how his stepfather got the job. Carlos had a long-term girlfriend whom he has known since the sixth grade. She broke up with him in December because he was starting to get interested in other girls. Carlos misses her and said that he is now sorry that his actions resulted in the relationship ending. He continues to be sexually active and stated that he always uses condoms because he does not want to get AIDS. Carlos has never impregnated any of his sexual partners.

Prior treatment: Carlos reported that he was on Ritalin for attention deficit hyperactivity disorder (ADHD) when he was younger but no longer takes that medication. He was seen for outpatient counseling at Child and Family Services. Carlos also saw a psychiatrist in North Kingstown whose name he could not remember. He has been on other psychotropic medications but does not know their names. Carlos has also been in "anger management classes all of my life."

Impressions

Carlos is a likable young man who was charming and engaging during the interview. He is a cognitively limited young man who is emotionally labile. His feelings are much more easily aroused and expressed than most of his peers. Carlos is aware of this with regard to his anger. He was candid in describing his serious and long-standing problems with impulse control and anger. Although Carlos was surprisingly open and self-disclosing in describing his temperament, he was concerned about how much information he was revealing and made several comments to that effect. For example, in discussing his marijuana use, Carlos stated: "You're not going to tell Br. Joe that I smoked marijuana?" I replied: "He probably knows." After the interview, we bumped into Br. Joe in the corridor. I mentioned this to him and he whispered to Carlos: "I already know."

Carlos admitted to his latest charges of assault and acknowledged that he has a very bad temper. Even as he described his problems with anger, there were subtle but observable changes in his eyes and posture. When I mentioned this to him, he commented: "Yeah, my eyes got bigger didn't they?" Carlos acknowledged that even after all the anger management training, he continues to have problems controlling his aggression. In his words, "I'm fine when I am in the class, but when I am in a situation, it doesn't work." Just about any sort of frustration or mild provocation can trigger his anger. Carlos denied experiencing any feelings of depression except under normal and appropriate circumstances, like when his girlfriend broke up with him. Although Carlos was previously diagnosed with a mood disorder and major depressive disorder, he does not report any signs or symptoms of a mood or depressive disorder at the present time. He has no history of past, recent, or current suicidal thoughts. Although he is not at risk of harming himself, he is at risk of harming others because of his poor impulse control and difficulty managing his anger. Carlos expressed mixed feelings about being at Ocean Tides for the summer. He is unhappy about being in custody but is grateful that he has not been sent back to the training school. Carlos is relieved that he is not being waived for trial as an adult for his recent charges.

DSM-IV Diagnosis:

312.82 Conduct Disorder, Adolescent Onset

314.01 Attention-Deficit/Hyperactivity Disorder, Combined Type (moderate to severe, by history)

305.20 Cannabis Abuse (in remission by virtue of incarceration)

Recommendations

Despite the considerable amount of anger management training that he has had, Carlos continues to need help in this area. The main problem he experiences is being able to apply this training in actual situations. Part of the problem is that Carlos does not recognize or anticipate what will trigger his anger. Prior cognitive testing indicated that his understanding of social situations and his knowledge of conventional standards of social behavior are limited and considerably below average. An approach that might help is to utilize more active role-playing and behavioral rehearsal to recreate the situations that instigate his loss of control. I would suggest identifying several concrete triggers and creating simulated situations in which he is repeatedly provoked until he can maintain control over his anger. This is an approach that has been successfully used to train riot police to maintain control even under extreme provocation and harassment. I discussed this with Carlos and he indicated that he would be willing to participate. A recent [date] neuropsychological evaluation documents Carlos's learning deficits and lists a number of helpful specific recommendations for use in the classroom.

EXAMPLE OF AN INTERVIEW WITH AN OPEN AND SELF-DISCLOSING RESIDENT

Clinical Psychological Evaluation

Name: Greg

Referral: Greg is a recently admitted resident at the Narragansett Campus of Ocean Tides. He was referred for a clinical psychological evaluation.

Behavioral observations: Greg is a 16-year-old Caucasian young man of average height and broad, muscular build. He has very short brown hair and was cleanly groomed. Greg was not wearing any earrings or other jewelry and has no visible scars, tattoos, or other distinguishing marks. He shook hands when I introduced myself and accompanied me without any hesitation. Greg was very outgoing and friendly. He was talkative, answered questions completely, and frequently offered additional information spontaneously. He was very open and self-disclosing. At times he returned to prior topics to add more details. Although Greg maintained direct eye contact at all times, he was very fidgety and restless. He spoke rapidly but clearly. Greg smiled often and his mood was generally very upbeat and positive. He expressed a range of emotions that were always appropriate to the content of the conversation. Greg did not express any unusual ideas or exhibit any behavior that was out of the ordinary or inappropriate. The evaluation was completed easily and successfully.

Interview

Family: Greg lives with his mother and two younger half brothers, aged 6 and 8 years, in West Warwick. His 19-year-old brother is in the Jobs Corps and lives in Exeter. Greg's parents divorced when he was about 5 years old. Greg said that he did not know why his parents divorced. His mother reported in a prior evaluation that her former husband abused alcohol and she had been a victim of repeated serious physical abuse by him. She also indicated that Greg had witnessed this abuse on multiple occasions. Greg's father, who is a carpenter, moved to Florida and Texas after the divorce but recently returned to Rhode Island so he could be closer to his sons. Greg reported that his father stayed in touch with him intermittently when he was living out of state. His mother had a common-law husband who lived with them for about 8 years. The two younger boys are from that relationship. Greg reported that she has had a new boyfriend for about a year. Greg is not close to his mother and stated plainly that he does not really like her very much. He indicated that she was out drinking almost every night with her boyfriend and often would not come in until 4 a.m. Greg had the responsibility of taking care of his two younger brothers. He said that she and her boyfriend have cut back on their drinking and she is around more. Although Greg indicated that he and his mother have been getting along better recently, he continues to have a lot of resentment toward her because of her past behavior. Greg's father has remarried. Greg might be interested in living with him but prefers to live independently when he is old enough.

Charges: Greg is in custody for robbery. He took two guns, a shotgun, and a .22-caliber rifle from an automobile. Greg also had prior charges of assault and conspiracy to commit armed robbery. Regarding the assault, he and another of our residents beat up the victim pretty badly, breaking his arm and a couple of ribs. When I asked how he was apprehended for the robbery, Greg replied: "Someone snitched." He indicated that he probably would not have been caught otherwise. Greg also has a number of disorderly conduct charges that he did not mention.

Substance use: Greg reported that he was a regular and heavy user of marijuana. He stated that he smoked every day, usually a couple of blunts. He acknowledged that he would have smoked even more if he could have afforded it. Greg also drinks alcohol and "likes the hard stuff." He said that he had reduced his intake of both marijuana and alcohol prior to entering the program.

Interests, plans for the future, and prior school adjustment: Greg is in the 11th grade, which is the appropriate grade level for him. He is not interested in sports and said that his main interest is his girlfriend. They have been dating for more than 2 years. If he has money, they will go to a movie or out to eat. Otherwise, they just hang out. Greg wants to return to W High School after he completes the program. After graduation, he wants to work for a couple of years and then go to college. He is still uncertain about career training. For example, he indicated that he wants to be a plumber but did not realize that it is not necessary to go to college to achieve that goal.

Prior treatment: Greg received treatment for ADHD several years ago at Kevin Carlos Mental Health. He had trials on Adderall and Concerta. His mother reported that she did not perceive any changes in his behavior when he was on the medication. Greg was only marginally compliant with the medication.

Impressions

Greg is a likable young man but clearly has great difficulty with impulse control. Greg has a long history of behavioral difficulties in school, including swearing at teachers and other related acting-out behavior. When provoked, Greg gets angry quickly and is likely to act without thinking. For example, he described an incident in which his mother was on his older brother's back. His brother tried to throw her off by turning around quickly. In the process he accidentally hit Greg in the face with his elbow. Even though Greg realized that it was unintentional, he got angry and punched a hole in the wall. What provokes Greg's anger is someone saying something bad about his girlfriend. When I asked him if he would get angry if someone made a negative comment about his mother, he said: "No, because I really don't like her that much." Once angered, it takes him about half an hour to calm down. Greg reported that he went through anger management training in the Key program and indicated that it was very helpful. He uses deep breathing and walking to calm himself. Greg said that he is not free to take a walk at Ocean Tides when he gets upset.

One of my concerns is Greg's lack of remorse for his behavior. For example, in describing his assault charge, he mentioned that he "messed him (the victim) up pretty bad." Not only did he show a lack of empathy or concern for his victim, but also his major concern was that his foot was sore from kicking the victim. Greg is very open and honest in expressing his opinions and is not concerned with political correctness. He stated in unequivocal terms that the local police do not like him and he does not like them, alleging that they are involved in a variety of illegal behaviors. Greg acknowledged that he has an attitude of belligerence and contempt toward the police and makes no effort to hide it. In short, he is an angry young man even though he appears outwardly as affable, outgoing, and personable.

Greg's major unresolved emotional issues are his resentment toward his mother and the residuals of having witnessed serious physical abuse as a child. While I did not ask him about this specifically because I did not know about it at the time of the interview, he did not mention it when I asked him about the reasons for his parent's divorce. He either does not remember witnessing the abuse or is denying it. Greg did not reveal any negative or mixed feelings about his father. Greg is not depressed and did not report or show any signs of a thought disorder or mood disorder. He has no past, recent, or current suicidal ideation or attempts. Prior cognitive testing indicated that Greg is functioning in the low average range of intelligence, between the 9th and 13th percentiles for youngsters his age.

DSM-IV Diagnosis:

312.82 Conduct Disorder, Adolescent-Onset Type

314.01 Attention-Deficit/Hyperactivity Disorder, Combined Type (by history)

305.00 Alcohol Abuse

305.20 Cannabis Abuse

Recommendations

Greg appears to be making a good initial adjustment to the program. Although he says that prior anger management training has been helpful, I do not think he is in control of his anger as much as he seems to think. Consequently, I recommend that he participate in the Anger Management Group at Ocean Tides. Greg harbors considerable resentment toward his mother and conflicted feelings toward his father that need to be addressed in individual counseling. If the description of his mother in a previous Diagnostic Assessment Services evaluation is accurate, family counseling may be difficult because of her distrustful and guarded behavior, denial of her prior substance abuse, and questionable motivation for cooperating and participating in treatment. In view of his volatile temper and avoidance types of defenses, these issues will have to be approached carefully and tactfully. In terms of his academics, Greg has been in special education for a long time and will require additional assistance. His plan to go to college is probably not realistic in view of his intelligence and academic history, but he could benefit from some vocational counseling while he is here. Although he wants to return to public high school when he completes the program, he is much more likely to be successful at the Providence Campus or a comparable program that offers smaller classes in a structured environment.

Index